What's Too Much,
What's Too Little, and
What's Just Right for You!

The
EXERCISE
BALANCE

PAULINE POWERS, MD & RON THOMPSON, PHD

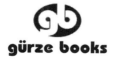

gürze books

The Exercise Balance
What's Too Much, What's Too Little, and What's Just Right for You!

Gürze Books, LLC
P.O. Box 2238
Carlsbad, CA 92018
(800) 756-7533
www.gurze.com

Cover design by Johnson Design
Illustrations by André Holmes

Library of Congress Cataloging-in-Publication Data

Powers, Pauline S.
   The exercise balance : what's too much, what's too little, and what's just right for you! / Pauline Powers & Ron Thompson.
      p. cm.
   Includes index.
   ISBN-13: 978-0-936077-02-4
   1. Exercise. 2. Exercise addiction. I. Thompson, Ron A. II. Title.
   RA781.P64 2008
   613.7'1--dc22
                        2008005135

The authors and publishers of this book intend for this publication to provide accurate information. It is sold with the understanding that it is meant to complement, not substitute for, professional medical and/or psychological services.

1 3 5 7 9 10 8 6 4 2

To my husband, Henry Powers, a constant source of encouragement.

—Pauline Powers

To my daughter, Allison, whose bicycle has often served her as a faithful companion.

To my good friend, Steve Gribble, whose ALS took away his beloved hiking and golf before it took him from us.

—Ron Thompson

Contents

List of Tables & Figures

Tables

Figures

Acknowledgments

We appreciate the time, energy, and thoughtful input from our editor and publisher, Leigh Cohn. André Holmes, medical illustrator, provided superb drawings to illustrate several points in the book. Roberta Sherman, PhD, colleague and friend, gave continuous support to the authors. Sherry McKnight, secretary extraordinaire, devoted many hours to helping us prepare the manuscript.

Introduction

We decided to write *The Exercise Balance* when we realized many of our family, friends, patients, and coworkers were exercising too much or too little. Some suffer from obesity and are sedentary, while others exercise obsessively, despite being dramatically underweight and physically ill. Also, although both of us exercise on a regular basis, we recognize how challenging it can be to achieve and maintain a healthy balance.

I, Pauline, a Professor of Psychiatry and Behavioral Medicine at the University of South Florida, have integrated moderate exercise into the treatment of obesity and eating disorders for over 30 years. I concluded that one way to increase the chances of living to a healthy, active old age is to exercise regularly, so I schedule exercise in the same way I schedule patient appointments. Since I don't particularly like strength exercise and fear that I wouldn't do do them on my own, I work with a physical trainer twice a week. I also belong to the YMCA and do aerobics three or four times a week for 30 minutes each time. Writing this book has also provided me with added motivation, but I realize that not everyone can use that approach!

From Ron: I'm a self-declared "sports nut," and for me the motivation for writing a book about balance is somewhat different. As a psychologist, I've specialized in athletes and eating disorders and have worked with sport groups such as the National Collegiate Athletic Association and the International Olympic Committee Medical Commission. Professionally, I've seen the negative consequences of overtraining, including physical illness and injury (and even death), destruction of family relationships, and the loss of promising careers. On a personal level, after having coronary bypass surgery several years ago, I had "a moment of clarity" and decided to become more physically active in order to avoid additional health problems. Since then, I have exercised regularly, running and doing resistance training. Recently, my physicians discovered that exercise had helped me to develop collateral vessels within my heart that have protected it from tissue damage due to an inadequate blood supply. Although I sometimes complain that I "hate running," my exercise program may have saved my life, and now I am even more motivated to both continue my workouts and to encourage others to do the same.

Between us, we have treated thousands of individuals at both ends of the exercise continuum and understand the importance of finding a balance. Today's society has what many consider to be "an obesity epidemic," yet ironically, there are also increased numbers of people engaging in extreme exercise, such as ultra-marathoners and eating disordered individuals with "activity anorexia." Each of these polar opposite groups have dangerous medical conditions, such as the diabetes and heart disease that underexercisers widely experience, and the musculoskeletal and cardiovascular problems which are common to overexercisers. These are two sides to the same coin—unhealthy activity levels. In this book, we provide in-depth descriptions of the characteristics and hazards of both extremes and specific steps to take towards moderation.

Our primary goal for *The Exercise Balance* is to offer practical information that can be used by most individuals—no matter where they fall along the activity continuum—to develop and maintain a balanced, healthy, and flexible exercise program. Our secondary goal is to accomplish this by presenting scientific research when available, anecdotal information when relevant, and personal accounts when informative and interesting. We also wanted to provide a user-friendly approach for those wishing to implement change, as well as useful guidelines for health care professionals, coaches, and trainers, who work with anyone from the chronically ill and inactive to athletes who push themselves obsessively.

Since both men and women are subject to the information in the text, we switch between the pronouns "he" and "she" from time to time, but in most cases we are writing about both genders. Also, we often address "you," the reader.

Whether you are in good general health, or suffer from physical illness or chronic disease, we want to stress that it is possible to achieve a healthy exercise balance at any age. Even if you have never participated in sports or in regular physical activity, you can add exercise and improve the chances of living a longer, healthier, more energetic life. If you have been active to the point of injury or illness, we will help you recognize compulsions and find the commitment to change.

How This Book Is Organized

The first two chapters define concepts such as balance, motivation to change, health and fitness, energy balance and weight, and the measurement of energy expenditure and physical activity. These are appropriate for all readers. The next few chapters of the book are particular to overexercisers *or* underexercisers, and although both are valuable for professionals, self-help readers need only use the parts that are appropriate to their situations. Chapter Eight focuses on specific guidelines based on age—which should be interesting for everyone—Chapter Nine has special considerations for individuals with chronic illnesses such as diabetes, high blood pressure, heart disease, osteoarthritis, obesity, eating disorders, and mental illness.

Given such a wide range of interests and audience, we have attempted to present a balanced text. There is a combination of scientific explanation, self-help advice, and instructions for professionals—physicians, therapists, dietitians, athletic trainers, physical therapists, and educators at every level. With so many types of readers, we have tried to make the language clear enough for everyone and with adequate depth for those who are interested in details. In many instances, we provide additional reading and websites for more information. For example, the video animations at the Centers for Disease Control and Prevention show how to perform certain exercises far more effectively than the written instructions we could provide. All of the Internet resources included in this book were current at the time of publication, but it is safe to assume that the sites will be updated over time. However, all of the sources are credible research and government institutions and should continue to be considered reliable.

Motivation

We will describe proven methods of improving motivation and maintaining the path to a healthy lifestyle, as well as pitfalls to avoid. Motivation for change depends on many factors that vary by age, health status, and circumstances. For example, today's children need to incorporate physical activity at an early age to offset the inordinate amount of time they spend in front of screens.

Obese adults may face life-threatening medical complications unless they become more active. And, in a relatively short period of time, the addition of stretching and mild strength exercises can improve vitality, mobility, and energy for older sedentary adults with health problems. Among the excessively active, athletes who abuse exercise and develop "overtraining" syndrome will be given tips on how to rejuvenate the body. In this situation coaches may be able to convince them to rest appropriately, and moderate the sport routine so that performance actually improves. This can be a powerful motivating factor in the context of increasing athletic performance.

One concern about the self-help format is that some readers may misinterpret and possibly misuse the information. For example, a few years ago when certain nutritionists recommended that people follow a "low fat" regimen, some individuals decided, "if low fat is good, then no fat must be better." We've seen some of them in our eating disorders practices. They eliminated as much fat as humanly possible, becoming obsessive in their thinking about dietary fat. They missed the nutritional value, satiety effect, and taste satisfaction that comes from a more balanced diet. Likewise, we've also treated patients who believed, "if some exercise is good, then more must be better," but this is not necessarily true. So, please take our recommendations on exercise as intended: moderate, flexible, and balanced strategies for therapeutic change. If you have specific concerns, please consult with your heath care providers and qualified fitness specialists.

CHAPTER 1

Exercise Balance

In this chapter, we introduce the idea of balance and explain why some people seem to gravitate to extremes. Both overexercisers and underexercisers have marked similarities, psychologically and physically. Finding balance requires integrating mind and body, and doing so leads to better health and a more rounded life. Eating and exercise are connected, and we will discuss how society is mired in an obesity epidemic as well as a fitness epidemic.

Balance is the perfect state of still water.
Let that be a model. It remains quiet within
And is not disturbed on the surface.
—Confucius

We are certainly not the first authors to address the concept of balance. While we would not aspire to the eloquence of the eminent Chinese philosopher Confucius or his contemporary, the Greek poet Euripides, who wrote, "The best and safest thing is to keep a balance in your life, acknowledge the great powers around us and in us," we can simply affirm that in exercise, balance is the key to good health. It is has been an ideal pursuit for centuries and is the central theme of this book.

We hope to convince you that moderation, flexibility, and balance are important to good health. We will provide tips on motivation and specific guidelines for a healthy exercise balance at any age. Whether you are in good general health or suffer from any of several physical illnesses, there are ways to safely increase your activity level and improve your vitality. Even if you have never participated in sports or in regular physical activity you can change and begin to feel better and improve your chances to live a healthier more energetic life. If you have been too active, you can learn the meaning behind this behavior and find the commitment to change to a more rewarding lifestyle.

Two Sides of the Same Coin

Although they may appear to be entirely disparate, there are actually similarities between people who are too physically active and those who are too sedentary. Besides the obvious observation that they are not taking care of their bodies, for both, physical health can be seriously impaired—although specific problems may not become apparent until later in life. For example, some female runners lose their menstrual periods and are at risk for bone loss. However, stress fractures associated with osteoporosis may not occur until they are much older. Among sedentary people, there is an increased chance of developing hardening of the arteries, technically called atherosclerosis; but they may not experience a heart attack until decades after this process has begun.

Another important consideration for people at either extreme is a disconnection between mind and body. For many centuries, the mind and body were considered separate but in the last 150 years this idea has been challenged, notably by Sigmund Freud, who in 1923 said, "...the ego is first and foremost a bodily ego."[1] The implication is that bodily states are influenced by the thinking, feeling part of the brain and vice versa. To achieve a healthy exercise balance, there needs to be a coming together of mind and body. When this integration does not occur, physical and psychological problems often result.

Patient Examples

Jennifer was a 17-year-old with anorexia nervosa. Despite being significantly underweight, she exercised two to three hours every day, regardless of the weather or her health. She felt that she had to exercise and became anxious and fearful when she didn't. Subsequently, she suffered three stress fractures during her senior year of high school, which eventually led to her referral for treatment. Through therapy, she came to realize that her excessive exercise and self-starvation were devices that she used to shield herself from unhappiness that resulted from a hidden trauma. She was literally trying to run away from her thoughts and to become invisible through her thinness.

Bill, a 42-year-old financial planner, was 50 pounds overweight and took a variety of medications to control his diabetes and high blood pressure. Even as a child, Bill was interested in business, but he shied away from sports because he was not particularly coordinated or athletic. His lifestyle relied heavily on coffee and cigarettes to keep his mind sharp, long working hours, business lunches, and large home-cooked meals by his wife, who was also overweight. His minimum of free time was spent with their three children, but he felt that he mainly contributed to their wellbeing by making money. He knew that he should lose weight and give up smoking, but up until the time of his triple bypass coronary surgery, he never even thought about exercise.

For both Jennifer and Bill, the mind and body were disconnected, which led to dire consequences. Neither of them readily acknowledged that their physical activity—or lack thereof—was particularly harmful. She kept her thoughts and emotions buried; his mind was always full of numbers. She obsessed about her body and he ignored his. Neither of them lived a life of balance.

Balance

Think about the word *balance*. It almost always has a positive connotation, suggesting equilibrium, stability, and equality. We balance the wheels of our cars to get a safer, more comfortable ride. We marvel at a gymnast's great balance. We balance our checkbooks and budgets to manage our finances. Dietitians extol the virtues of a balanced diet. *Exercise*, like balance, is a concept that almost always has a positive connotation. Even people who do not exercise probably view the *idea* of exercise as a good thing.

When we speak of balance, we are not talking about a delicate one. Nor do we mean a single center point as opposed to an extreme. Rather, we are speaking of a broader, flexible, more comfortable mid-*range*. Depending on your needs and circumstances at a particular time, it may be more conducive or prudent to slide from near the center to a point within an acceptable range in either direction.

Balance appears to be such a worthwhile concept that it is puzzling why everyone would not choose or seem to want it. How can this be? Certainly some individuals have compulsive personalities or troubled emotions that lead or push them to extremes. There are also people who tend toward "all-or-nothing" thinking and typically see only black and white categories when making decisions. They don't even consider the middle ground. Some people may actually feel more physically or psychologically comfortable at an extreme. How is this possible?

First, they may spend so much time at one extreme that it actually feels normal and therefore comfortable. For instance, compulsive exercisers are like addicts and become anxious and upset by skipping a workout. For them, their obsessive behavior is the norm. In fact, taking a more balanced position would feel uneasy, at least for a while. Most excessive exercisers probably view their activity level as balanced, but that is just an illusion. They *need* to burn calories, relax their overtaxed mind, or stay competitive, because they enjoy it so much and have difficulty setting limits. They believe "more must be better." We see this cognitive distortion repeatedly with anorexic patients who are unable to accurately see their own devastating thinness. They perceive fat where there is none. In the same manner, excessive exercisers neither acknowledge nor realize the damage they are doing to their bodies. Similarly, underexercisers may have been inactive for so long that a sedentary lifestyle is what's normal for them—anything more active would be unfamiliar to them. However, at some level, most overexercisers and underexercisers probably know that their behavior is not normal, healthy, or balanced.

> Most overexercisers and underexercisers probably know that their behavior is not normal, healthy, or balanced.

Another reason is that, even though some people might acknowledge that balance in general is good, they may actually be afraid of it. Overexercisers may fear that they won't get as much satisfaction from working out less or may end up not exercising at all. People with eating disorders often look at weight gain with the same kind of "all-or-nothing" thinking. They fear that if they begin to gain weight, they won't be able to stop. They envision themselves like giant balloons being over-inflated. These individuals are in essence afraid of losing control. Likewise, excessive exercisers may feel out of control if they do not continue with their routine. People who don't exercise regularly—or at all—equally resist upsetting their habits. Someone like Bill, from our previous example, may worry about creating a financial burden from working less; or, given a lack of familiarity with athletics, may fear failure.

Some people may prefer an extreme because they equate balance with being "in the middle." They balk at this idea because it would mean they are "average," and they do not want to be "average" in any aspect of their lives. They resist the idea of "being like everyone else." As long as they are at an extreme, they view themselves as "special" or at least more noticeable. Nowhere is this more evident than in "ultra-endurance" sports—the Badwater Ultramarathon is a prime example. This 135-mile race starts at the lowest point in the United States in Death Valley and finishes near the summit of Mt. Whitney, the highest point in the contiguous states. To make matters worse, it is run during the hottest part of summer, where the monthly average temperature can reach 117° and the nation's hottest day on record occurred at 134° on July 10, 1913. Some competitors have run the course back and forth and even more. Could any physical contest possibly be *more* extreme? Yet, it is precisely the extreme nature of these competitions that draws more and more participants every year. What must it take to prepare for a race like that? Besides the wear and tear on the body, imagine the sacrifices that would need to be made with regard to work, relationships, and other interests.

Many people who strive to be number one in a sport may find it difficult to believe that it is possible to excel in athletic pursuits and still have a rounded life. Therefore, we present the inspirational story of Roger Bannister, the first person to run a mile in under four minutes.

In his autobiography,[2] Bannister portrays himself as being a tense and excitable boy who ran to get from place to place, as a solitary endeavor, and to escape bullies. At Oxford, "where a man without a sport is like a ship without a sail," he took up running because he had little aptitude for ball games. The descriptions of his undergraduate life indicated that, "running took only a small part of my time," and although he trained diligently, his life was filled with studies, developing friendships, and being active in the organization of athletic clubs, to which "running took second place." After graduation, he continued to compete at a very high level and devoted himself to scientifically researching how to increase breathing during exercise, which got him interested in medicine. He took breaks from competition traveling the countryside, walking, climbing, swimming, and sleeping in the open. During these excursions, when he ran, it was purely for enjoyment. In early preparation for the 1952 Olympics, he abandoned cross-country racing, never ran for longer than a half an hour, and didn't time himself with a stopwatch.

As a medical student, his time for running was even more limited. Leading up to the Olympic Games, he avoided serious races and, "saw no useful purpose in exhausting myself needlessly." His method of training, which was far different than his peers, was to not overextend himself but to remain fresh. The press criticized his methods when he failed to win a medal at the Olympics in Helsinki, even though he broke the world's record in the 1,500 meters and finished in fourth place, less than a second behind the winner. Afterwards, his hospital work became so pressing that he nearly stopped running entirely.

As he prepared himself for the assault on the four-minute mile, which in 1954 was one of the most revered goals in all of sport, Bannister maintained the same approach to training. He applied what he had studied about oxygen consumption in order to run at peak intensity for a longer stretch, but he still practiced moderation. During a typical week of hard workouts, he made it a point to take some days off to reinvigorate his muscles. He also didn't participate in any races for eight months, storing up his competitive energy. On the historic day, he lunched with friends and their children to calm his nerves. With the support of teammates who paced him, they "shared a place where no man had yet ventured—secure for all time."

We presented so much of Roger Bannister's story to illustrate a few points. First, it shows that it is possible to achieve extreme athletic success without overtraining and excluding other aspects of your life. Second, his training methods speak volumes about the value of not overdoing it. And, finally, his life, while filled with high achievement is the perfect example of balance. In fact, he's as recognized for his distinguished career as a neurologist—for which he was knighted by the Queen of England—as for his "Dream Mile."

Weight & Fitness

Everyone knows that our culture has an "Overweight Epidemic," but it is also plagued by a *fitness epidemic*. Most Americans weigh too much and exercise too little, and there is an obvious connection between the two. Weight is influenced by a variety of factors: heredity, age, metabolic rate, calories consumed, and activity level. When someone takes in more calories than are utilized, that person may not gain a lot of weight according to these factors. For example, if a person's parents were both naturally thin, they are unlikely to ever be overweight. However, most people don't fall into this group, and for the masses over consumption of calories and lack of exercise leads to weight gain.

There are several relationships between eating and exercise. For example, exercise uses the energy that has been provided by the foods we eat. Eating restores the energy used by exercise. Some people might intentionally exercise to "compensate" for what they have eaten. Others may eat so much that they don't feel capable of being active. Eating disorder patients often are apt to overexercise and undereat, especially when it comes to consuming fats. Recent research on eating disorders and genetics suggests that a disturbance in a neurotransmitter—the brain chemical called serotonin—creates a vulnerability to developing an eating disorder that can be triggered by dieting or exercise.[3,4] There is also a connection between underexercising and overeating, both of which contribute to obesity. This topic is explained more fully in Chapter Six.

Today's society promotes poor eating and exercise habits. In the past few decades, there has been an abundant availability of high-fat, high-calorie, processed foods. The fast food industry aggressively markets "super sized" portions that are loaded with calories from sweeteners and fat, which makes the food taste good. Advertising is aimed at youngsters, who develop lifelong eating preferences, and there has been an avalanche in these kinds of restaurants. In 1968, there were about 1,000 McDonalds outlets, and by 2002 there were more than 30,000,[5] besides which there are now thousands of different brands of fast food—with 95% of Americans partaking at least once in a while. In a 2003 Gallup Poll, 31% indicated that they eat fast food weekly, and 21% said they have it several times per week.[6] Consider that an average-sized man exceeds his recommended daily calorie intake with only one meal at McDonalds by consuming a Big Mac˚, order of large fries, and a super-sized milk shake. Factor in that in the past few decades, physical activity has decreased. Computers have placed much of the job force behind desks and far fewer people do work that requires much energy expenditure. This combination of poor eating and limited movement results in obesity.

As obesity increases in a country, eating disorders also becomes more common. This means that not only is a large segment of society sedentary, but another, perhaps smaller, segment of society adopts unhealthy dietary restriction and excessive exercise as a means of coping with the fear of obesity. This may occur because as the medical community and general society emphasize the real dangers of obesity, there is a tendency to glamorize or admire people who participate in sports or who maintain a low weight. Unfortunately, this glamorization by the media and advertising serves to shift the focus from health to appearance. Thus, many individuals become more concerned—or even obsessed—with trying to meet an unrealistic standard for thinness than they are for physical and psychological health.

Despite the obstacles, it is possible to moderate eating and physical activity to a healthy level. Attempting to change behavior in only one these areas—such as simply dieting to lose weight—is usually futile. As far as eating, we generally recommend following the Food Pyramid and dietary guidelines developed by the USDA. This information is available at their excellent, interactive website, www.mypyramid.gov. Otherwise, for specific concerns, we suggest consulting with a registered dietitian.

In this book, we are primarily interested in helping to determine how much to exercise. For people who are overdoing it, we will discuss the harmful consequences and provide guidelines for moderation. For those who are just beginning to exercise or feel the need to do more, we will explain what steps to take. Balanced exercise is the key; and, we will describe proven methods of improving motivation for change and maintaining a healthy physical activity routine for life.

Notes

1. *a bodily ego.* Freud S: *The Ego and the Id.* WW Norton & Co., New York, 1960.

2. *In his autobiography.* Bannister R: *The Four-Minute Mile: fiftieth-Anniversary Edition.* Lyons Press, Guilford, CT, 2004.

3. *dieting or exercise.* Kaye WH, Guido FK, Meltzer DD, Price JC, McConaha CW, Crossan PJ, Klump KL, Rhodes L: Altered serotonin 2A receptor activity in women who have recovered from bulimia nervosa. *American Journal of Psychiatry 158:1152-1155, 2001.*

4. *triggered by dieting and/or exercise.* Kaye WH, Barbarich KP, Gendall KA, Ferstrom J, Fernstrom M, McConaha CW, Kishore A: Anxiolytic effects of acute tryptophan depletion in anorexia nervosa. *International Journal of Eating Disorders 33:257-267, 2003.*

5. *more than 30,000.* Schlosser E: *Fast Food Nation.* Penguin Books, New York, 2002.

6. *several times per week.* Gallup G: *The Gallup Poll.* Rowman and Littlefield, Lanham, MD. 2003.

CHAPTER 2

Exercise Explained

In this chapter, we describe and discuss exercise and associated concepts such as physical activity, physical fitness, metabolic fitness, personal health, energy regulation, and body weight. These are terms that are used throughout this book. We also briefly discuss how physical activity and energy output are measured. We begin with some definitions of these concepts, as well as describe the relationships between and among them.

Most people think of exercise as a planned activity that is performed on a track or in a gym, or referred to as "working out," such as running, weight lifting, step aerobics, or calisthenics. Exercise can be defined in many ways, but for our purposes we prefer a broader definition such as the one proposed by Knuttgen,[1] who designates exercise as "any activity involving the generation of force by activated muscles, including activities of daily living, work, recreation, and competitive sports."

Scientists have determined that there are two general types of exercise—aerobic and anaerobic. Simply put, *aerobic* means "with oxygen" and *anaerobic* means "without oxygen." Exercise can be described as aerobic or anaerobic based not only on the type of activity but also its intensity and duration. *Intensity* describes how hard an individual exercises and *duration* indicates how long. Exercise balance involves moderating both intensity and duration to produce a healthy but flexible regimen of physical activity, given one's particular needs and health status. The combination of the two is the foundation of exercise balance.

Aerobic vs. Anaerobic Exercise

Even though a distinction can be made between aerobic and anaerobic exercise, they are not mutually exclusive. Most exercise is neither entirely aerobic nor anaerobic and, in actuality, involves *both*. How much a particular type of exercise is one or the other depends upon its type, intensity, and duration. The first few minutes tend to be anaerobic, regardless of the type of activity—whether you are running, doing push-ups, or working in your garden. The body can automatically shift from anaerobic to aerobic metabolism with the primary difference being the amount of energy that is produced and how it is provided. Both aerobic and anaerobic exercise burn calories, but high intensity exercise will usually burn more. Lower intensity usually burns fewer calories with a greater proportion apt to be from fat. Anaerobic exercise tends to build more muscle, which increases metabolism.

Exercise that is considered primarily aerobic typically involves activities that are sustained at lower intensities for greater duration, such as jogging, bicycling, and swimming. If enough fuel and oxygen are available, the body can continue aerobic exercise for long periods of time, especially as one's conditioning and fitness improve. Not surprisingly, the body's need for oxygen increases proportionate to exercise intensity. At some point during aerobic exercise, the body's need for oxygen is too great for it to be met by aerobic metabolism alone. It then must rely, at least in part, on anaerobic metabolism.

> Aerobic exercise is generally less intense than anaerobic exercise and performed for longer periods of time.

Anaerobic exercise primarily involves activities that are of higher intensity but shorter duration, where energy is consumed in spurts, such as lifting weights, sprinting, or playing football. As mentioned previously, anaerobic means without oxygen. This does not mean that oxygen is unimportant or not involved in anaerobic exercise. Rather, it means that anaerobic exercise does not require that *increased* oxygen be delivered to the muscles that are being used. It also means that although less energy is produced than in the aerobic metabolic process, it is produced faster. Because of this diminished energy production and lactic acid build-up (related to fatigue), a person can perform anaerobic exercise for only short periods of time.

Aerobic and anaerobic exercise not only rely on different energy systems, they also utilize different muscle fibers. Aerobic exercise primarily involves Type I, or slow contraction speed, twitch muscle fibers. Anaerobic exercise primarily involves Type II, or fast contraction speed, twitch fibers. There are two types of Type II fibers, Type IIa and Type IIb. All people have a mix of muscle fibers but most people have more of one type than another.

An individual's muscle fiber content is believed to be genetically determined. To compensate for this, different sports employ various training approaches to produce adaptations in Type I or II muscle fibers. For example, distance runners like to increase the aerobic capabilities of their Type I fibers to boost cardiovascular fitness, whereas football players may want to increase the anaerobic capabilities of their Type II fibers to enhance strength, a particular skill, and/or agility. It should be noted that certain illnesses are associated with changes in the proportion of muscle fiber types. Diabetic patients are known to have more Type IIb fibers and fewer Type I fibers. This may account for some of the difficulty diabetics experience with aerobic, or endurance, exercise.

TABLE 2.1. Characteristics of Muscle Fiber Types

	Aerobic	Anaerobic	
Main Fiber Type	Type I	Type IIa	Type IIb
Contraction Time	slow	fast	very fast
Activity	aerobic	longer-term anaerobic	shorter-term anaerobic
Group with higher proportion of fiber type	long-distance runners	sprinters	diabetics

Both Type IIa and Type IIb fibers have fast contraction speeds but Type IIb fibers are faster than Type IIa. One reason that patients with diabetes mellitus may find aerobic, or endurance, exercise difficult is because they have a higher proportion of Type IIb muscle fibers.

What is the best type of exercise for you? It depends on your goals. For most individuals, we recommend a balanced approach that utilizes both aerobic and anaerobic metabolism to enhance strength as well as cardiovascular fitness and general health.

Physical Activity

Many different terms are used to describe exercise, one of which is *physical activity*. Distinctions can be made between exercise that is considered "planned behavior" and what has been termed "spontaneous physical activity,"[2] but we are interested in "physical activity," whether planned or spontaneous.

As mentioned earlier, we like Knuttgen's broad definition in which *all* physical activities, not just those involved in sports or at the local gym, are considered exercise. We also endorse Corbin and Lindsey's[3] more refined approach. They make the distinction between *exercise* (which includes "physical activity done for the purpose of getting physically fit") and lifestyle physical activity (which includes the many aspects of daily life, like raking leaves, shoveling snow, mowing grass, and climbing stairs). Additionally, the National Athletic Trainers Association[4] defines physical activity as consisting of "athletic, recreational or occupational activities that require physical skills and utilize strength, power, endurance, speed, flexibility, range of motion or agility."

Physical Fitness

According to the American College of Sports Medicine (ACSM),[5] *physical fitness* is defined as "the ability to perform moderate to vigorous levels of physical activity without undue fatigue and the capability of maintaining this capacity throughout life." Most experts agree that it is composed of five key elements: cardiorespiratory health (aerobic endurance), muscular endurance, muscular strength, flexibility, and body composition.

Interestingly, many sports experts, including Timothy Noakes, author of *The Lore of Running*,[6] believe that some people, such as elite athletes, need less training to become physically fit due to their outstanding genetics. Clearly these individuals have a unique advantage over most of the rest of us. Nevertheless, even if it takes more effort to become physically fit, the ultimate goal is overall health through a balanced approach.

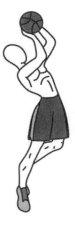

Five Components of Physical Fitness[7]

1. Cardiorespiratory or Aerobic Endurance

The ability to do moderately strenuous activity over a period of time. It reflects how well your heart and lungs work together to supply oxygen to your body during exertion and exercise. It is also called aerobic fitness.

2. Muscular Endurance

The ability to hold a particular position for a sustained period of time or repeat a movement many times. This could be the capability required to hold a two-pound weight above your head for five minutes or the effort required to lift that weight 20 consecutive times.

3. Muscular Strength

The ability to exert maximum force, such as lifting the heaviest weight you can budge, one time. It is possible to have muscular strength in one area, say your arms, while lacking strength in another area, such as your legs.

4. Flexibility

The ability to move a joint through its full range of motion or the elasticity of the muscle. This is how limber or supple you are.

5. Body Composition

The proportion of fat in your body compared to your bone and muscle. It does not refer to your weight in pounds or your shape.

Metabolic Fitness

What fitness means can differ depending on an exerciser's goals.[8] In a survey reported in *TIME* magazine,[9] it is curious to note that most people described themselves as "physically fit," even though half of those surveyed admitted to being overweight. *Can* you be fit and fat? Some medical and exercise scientists believe the answer is a resounding "yes!"—a notion popularized by Glenn Gaesser in his book, *Big Fat Lies*.[10] Gaesser presents compelling evidence that overweight individuals can improve certain aspects of their health (e.g., lowered blood pressure) through proper eating and moderate exercise *without* significantly reducing their weight. Gaesser emphasizes *metabolic fitness* rather than cardiorespiratory, and suggests changing the goal from being thin to healthy. He believes that metabolic fitness is a more reasonable goal because it promotes physical activity which, in his view, is under most people's control as opposed to cardiorespiratory fitness, which is often related to genetics.

The concept of metabolic fitness was first introduced by Jean-Pierre Després and colleagues,[11] who believe that increasing physical activity can reduce the onset of diabetes mellitus and cardiovascular disease. Their *metabolic syndrome* describes risk factors, such as abdominal or visceral obesity, and high blood pressure. Després[12] suggests that our sedentary lifestyle is "toxic" to the metabolic health of obese patients because it includes too many foods that upset a positive energy balance, causing obese people to continually ingest more calories than are burned. Rather than focusing on a reduction in weight, however, he recommends a healthy and balanced diet with less fat and refined sugar, and increased daily physical activity.

Also, according to Gaesser, metabolic fitness is about insulin or, more accurately, *insulin resistance*—a problem often associated with diabetes mellitus. He, like Després, believes that this condition can be decreased through healthy eating and physical activity.

Health vs. Fitness

You may be wondering how health and fitness differ and if you can have one without the other. Corbin and Lindsey define health as "…optimal well-being that contributes to the quality of life."[13] According to the ACSM, the quantity of exercise that is necessary to attain health benefits may differ from those for fitness. Lower levels of exercise may be sufficient to improve health, but not fitness.[14] That is, you can be healthy without being physically fit. An example would be my friend, Wade, who is 45 years old and is in good health, slightly overweight (BMI=27) and walks about 20 minutes at a time two or three days a week. He runs a successful business, has a happy home life, and enjoys many extracurricular activities. He is healthy but not physically fit. It is, of course, also possible to be healthy and physically fit.

But can a person be physically fit without being healthy? The answer is no. In order to be physically fit, one must first be healthy. Additionally, health is necessary to sustain physical fitness. The fact that a person can exercise does not necessarily imply fitness. Despite being malnourished and quite ill, many of our eating disorder patients exercise excessively. They are certainly not healthy, and their activity is not an indicator of fitness; rather, it is a compulsion fueled by anxiety and hyperactivity. Another example would be an accomplished athlete who does not eat enough to adequately fuel her physical activity and develops menstrual irregularities through a process known as low energy availability. As a consequence, she may experience bone loss and suffer fractures. If her unhealthy state is not corrected, it will eventually erode some of the components necessary for physical fitness, such as muscular strength, muscular endurance, and flexibility.

Regulation of Energy Balance and Weight

Understanding the way exercise influences weight and health requires an appreciation of the concept of *energy balance,* which the body maintains through a series of complicated systems. This means that the food we eat (energy in) minus the calories we use (energy out) either maintains, increases, or decreases our weight.

calories eaten = calories used = maintains weight
calories eaten > calories used = increases weight
calories eaten < calories used = decreases weight

Physical activity results in calories being used, but is only one of three important factors. Another is *basal metabolic rate* which is the number of calories required to keep the body operating while at rest and accounts for the majority of energy used in most people. A third factor is called *non-exercise adaptive thermogenesis,* which involves the calories required to digest and process food, termed the *thermic effect* of food. On the following page Figure 2.1 shows the way in which calories (energy out) are expended in most people.

FIGURE 2.1. Energy Expenditure

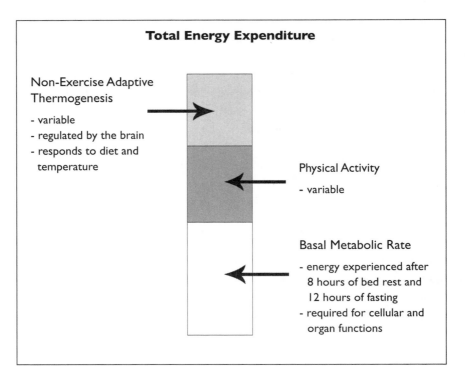

Physical activity accounts for a minority of daily calories used (energy out) and includes the basic activities of daily life (e.g., walking or getting out of a chair) and planned exercise (e.g., running or lifting weights). Basal metabolic rate (also called obligatory energy expenditure) accounts for the calories used to keep your body functioning, or the calories used when you are at rest. Non-exercise adaptive thermogenesis refers to the calories used to maintain fundamental activities (e.g. keeping your body warm or processing the food you eat). Used with permission from Yager J, Powers PS, *Clinical Manual of Eating Disorders*, p. 258, American Psychiatric Publishing, Inc., Washington, D.C., 2007.

The concept of energy balance is actually a bit more complex than it may initially appear because other factors are involved. As many of us know from firsthand experience, metabolism tends to decrease with age. Also, metabolic rate tends to increase with musculature. This means that, on average, males tend to have a metabolic rate that is about 10% higher than females because male bodies tend to have a greater proportion of muscle tissue. Recent research suggests that this inequity may be further increased by the fact that physical exercise usually results in a greater weight loss for men than for women.[15]

It may be surprising to learn that the majority of the population maintains a relatively stable weight when the range of possible—but not necessarily healthy—weight is from about 50 to 500 pounds. For example, a female anorexia nervosa patient who is 4'11" and weighs 50 pounds may be physically active even though she is semi-starved with multiple cardiac and orthopedic problems. On the other hand, a man who is 6'5" and weighs 500 pounds may have diabetes mellitus and high blood pressure but still be able to perform daily activities. These extreme examples are uncommon (and associated with severe medical problems) but life may still be supported for long periods of time. The reason most people's weight doesn't fluctuate (although it might be above or below what they think of as *ideal*) is because there are powerful biological systems at work. The part of the brain that regulates and coordinates the various factors that influence energy balance (e.g., appetite) is the hypothalamus (see Figure 2.2) which evolved to its current state over thousands of years and is relatively impervious to change. Therefore, the recent increase in overweight and obese people is not related to a change in brain functions. Instead, it is most probably related to the *decrease* in activity levels for most people in the modern world and the *increase* in the amount and availability of tasty high-fat and high-carbohydrate foods.[16, 17]

FIGURE 2.2. Hypothalamus

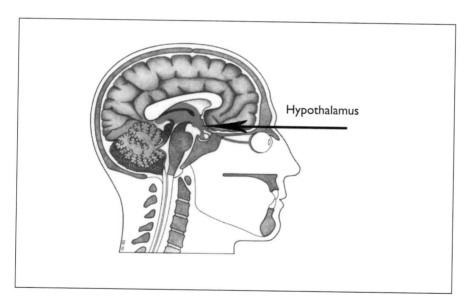

Hypothalamus

In terms of evolution, the "oldest" part of the brain includes the hypothalamus, which is a very important part of the system that regulates how many calories we eat as well as how many we use during physical activity to keep the body functioning. Most of the processes in this system function automatically.

Energy Availability Theory

A related concept is *energy availability*,[18] or dietary energy intake (calories eaten) minus exercise energy expenditure (calories used). According to this theory, low energy availability occurs when the total number of calories used in a day is greater than the total number of calories consumed. If this condition is severe and persistent, serious reproductive abnormalities can result. This imbalance is what might cause a female athlete to stop menstruating.

Although some experts think that marked changes in body composition (especially a lowered percentage of body fat) or low weight may also cause loss of menstrual periods in some female athletes, the theory of energy availability is different. This theory says that even though body weight and body fat might be low, an athlete's menstrual cycles will continue to be normal if she consumes enough calories to balance the amount of calories she expends during exercise. This concept explains why some underweight women maintain normal menstrual function and others do not.

Weight Issues

Another aspect of energy balance involves some of the myriad misconceptions that abound regarding weight loss, misconceptions that are continuously and intentionally promoted by the weight-loss industry and the popular press. As previously explained, weight cannot be defined or explained in simple terms. Losing weight does not just involve "will power," but rather is affected by several variables beyond how much one does or does not eat. Activity level, body composition, age, genetics, metabolism, set point, etc., all play a role.

Eating, in turn, is affected by several factors including neurobiology (e.g., neurotransmitters, neuropeptides), social learning, diet, psychological issues (anxiety, depression, obsessions, compulsions), environmental cues (e.g., availability of food), familial/social/cultural expectations (e.g., traditional or holiday foods), and certain medications, not to mention sheer hunger. For those of you whose primary concern is weight loss, we recommend (and Gaesser suggests)[19] that you focus on improving your health and fitness rather than just trying to reduce your weight. Too much focus on body size can lead to unhealthy dietary restrictions and obsessive thinking. In addition to using this book to help design a reasonable, regular exercise program, please consider consulting with a dietitian to create an appropriate meal plan. Additionally, working with a therapist can assist in reducing any dysfunctional, non-hunger-based eating.

Measurement of Energy Expenditure

Although there are several ways to determine energy expenditure, the most convenient method for the average person is self-reporting. Typically, the individual records his/her activities during a specified period of time. Using standard estimates of the energy expenditure for different activities, a total is derived by calculating the energy cost for each one. These standard estimates are called *metabolic equivalents*, or METs. One MET equals a metabolic rate consuming 3.5 ml. of oxygen per kilogram of body weight per minute, or in layman's terms, the energy (oxygen) used by the body as you sit quietly.

A MET is based on an individual's *resting energy expenditure*, or REE. If an activity uses three times the REE, then the activity has a MET of 3.0. The number of METs increases with the type, duration, and intensity of a given activity and is affected by weight and body composition. For example, a 150-pound person who shovels snow, a 6.0 MET activity, for 30 minutes would burn twice as many calories as he would while doing a 3.0 MET activity, like bowling, for the same amount of time. A heavier person would burn more calories in both activities.

A tracking guide for use of the MET system is available online.[20] It can be used to estimate the METs associated with everything from household chores to occupations to specific sports. Remember, though, unless you have had your personal REE determined in a performance laboratory, it is an *estimate,* as is the amount of energy used (calories burned) to perform a particular activity.

A similar method of determining energy expenditure was developed by Harris and Benedict[21] and uses *resting metabolic rate* (RMR) and a *physical activity factor* (PAF). The RMR is the energy needed to maintain necessary bodily functions. The PAF involves the intensity of activity. See Table 2.2 on the following page for instructions on how to calculate energy expenditure estimate using this method.

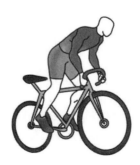

TABLE 2.2. How to Calculate the Number of Calories an Adult Needs to Maintain Weight—With and Without Activity

Directions: This is a two-step process. Using the Harris-Benedict Formula, first estimate your basal metabolic rate (BMR), which is the amount of calories your body needs to maintain its weight without activity. Once you determine your BMR, you then multiply it by your activity level factor (see Activity Factor Table) to estimate the number of calories needed to maintain weight with activity. Note that a different formula is given for each gender because of the differences between the male and female body.

Male formula

66 + (6.23 x weight in pounds) + (12.7 x height in inches) − (6.8 x age in years)

Note: The number "66" is a constant which is used in the calculation for all males.

Example

Ted is a 35-year-old male computer programmer who is 6'0" (72 inches) tall and weighs 185 pounds. He is in good health but wants to exercise moderately 3-5 times per week in an effort to improve his health markers (i.e., lower blood pressure and cholesterol levels).

Step One

185 pounds x 6.23 = 1152.55
72 inches x 12.7   =   914.40
35 years by 6.8   =   238.00
Now insert these numbers into the Harris-Benedict equation:
66 + 1152.55 + 914.40 − 238.00 = 1894.95 (estimated basal metabolic rate)

Step Two

Now multiply 1894.95 by the **activity factor** for the **moderately active level**, which is 1.55 = **2937.17 calories**. Theoretically, Ted needs **2900 calories** to maintain his weight with moderate exercise. Remember that this is an estimate. If Ted wants to lose weight, he would need to consume fewer calories and/or increase his exercise.

Female formula

655 + (4.35 x weight in pounds) + (4.7 x height in inches) − (4.7 x age in years)

Note: The number "655" is a constant which is used in the calculation for all females.

Example

Maria is a 20-year-old female athlete who is 5'5" (65 inches) tall and weighs 120 pounds. She competes on her college soccer team and trains hard 6 days per week. She wants to maintain her weight in order to feel strong when she competes. Thus, Maria needs to know approximately how many daily calories she needs in order to maintain her weight at her current training level.

Step One

120 pounds x 4.35 = 522
65 inches x 4.7   = 305.5
20 years x 4.7   = 94

Now insert these numbers into the Harris-Benedict equation:

655 + 522 + 305.5 – 94 = 1388.5 (estimated basal metabolic rate)

Step Two

Now multiply 1388.5 by the **activity factor** for the **very active level**, which is 1.725 = **2395.16 calories**. Theoretically, Maria needs about **2400 calories** each day to maintain her weight at her current training level. Remember that this is an estimate. If she increased her exercise, Maria would need to increase her caloric intake to maintain her weight.

TABLE 2.3. Activity Factor Table—Harris-Benedict Formula

Activity Level	Example Activities	Activity Factor
Sedentary	Little or no exercise	1.2
Lightly active	Light exercise 1-3 days/week	1.375
Moderately active	Moderate exercise 3-5 days/week	1.55
Very active	Hard exercise 6-7 days /week	1.725
Extra active	Very hard exercise/train 2x/day	1.9

Harris, JA,, & Benedict, FG. *A Biometric Study of Basal Metabolism in Man.* Washington DC, Carnegie Institute of Washington, 1919.

For anyone looking to lose weight, attempting to count—even believing that you *can* count—every calorie consumed is not only unrealistic, but also unnecessary. It can become an obsession and lead to other problems. Rather than focusing on calories and weight, focus on increasing physical activity while eating better to improve health.

Measurement of Physical Activity

One of the primary goals of this book is to help you find a healthy balance in your physical activity. If you want to make a change, it is useful to first assess your behavior, which in this case would be patterns of physical activity. Exercise assessments usually focus on the type, intensity, frequency, and duration, and can be quite technical and sophisticated. In performance laboratories, exercise scientists use ergometers (sophisticated exercise machines that measure the amount of work done by muscles) to measure precise exercise parameters and quantify exercise. They use terms like "force" (what changes state of rest or motion), "torque" (the effectiveness of force overcoming inertia), "work" (the force expressed through displacement), and "power" (the rate of performing work).[22] This type of evaluation is appropriate for research purposes and training elite athletes, but is beyond the needs of the average person. Assessments that are acceptable but less expensive and available to virtually everyone are actually more suitable for our purposes.

Exercise Machines

Some exercise machines, like treadmills, function in a fashion similar to the more sophisticated ergometers found in laboratories. Many home and gym exercise machines provide useful information, such as heart rate, estimates of calories burned, and accumulated exercise time. Additionally, many allow for a change in exercise intensity by increasing or decreasing resistance or speed. In general, these machines are a good choice for most people who want to quantify their current health and fitness levels and monitor progress in achieving their goals.

Self-Report Measures

Self-report inventories and questionnaires are frequently used because of their availability and low cost. However, measures of this type are subject to bias and unreliability precisely because they depend on the honesty and accuracy of the information provided by the subject—that's *you*! So keep it honest.

Many of these self-report measures now evaluate exercise in broader terms, looking at not only sports and planned exercise, but also at leisure time and work-related activities. Some also take into consideration the age of the person being surveyed. You can search the Web for special inventories for children and adolescents (e.g., the Self-

Administered Physical Activity Checklist),[23] adults (e.g., the Minnesota Leisure Time Physical Activity Questionnaire),[24] and older adults (e.g., the Physical Activity Scale for the Elderly).[25] Excessive exercise has become such a problem that there are now questionnaires that specialize in this area. (Further information about excessive exercise and related questionnaires are offered in Chapter Three.)

Heart Rate Monitors

The use of a heart rate monitor has become a popular and somewhat sophisticated way to evaluate exercise or, more importantly, how the body *reacts* to exercise. Most consist of a chest strap with a monitor and a device worn on the arm that displays your heart rate—many marathon runners wear them. Heart rate increases as exercise intensifies and a monitor of this kind can be used to help maintain a heart rate that is recommended or within a target range. Target ranges may be prescribed by a physician for a patient who is recovering from an ailment or disease, or chosen for a training regimen in which the individual maintains a certain heart rate to develop cardiovascular fitness. Although one's resting heart rate decreases with increased fitness, a low heart rate does not necessarily mean a person is fit. For example, some people who have anorexia nervosa have such low heart rates that they can prove to be lethal.

Pedometers

Another popular way to measure physical activity is with a pedometer, a device that senses the body's movements and counts the number of steps taken during an activity or throughout the day. A recommended and beneficial way to use a pedometer is to wear it and go about your business as usual, not giving thought to the device as it records the number of steps taken. After a week or two, average the daily totals to determine your approximate number of steps per day. Once your fitness or health goals are determined (perhaps with the help of a physician or trainer) you can adjust the number of steps needed to meet personal goals.

Some people might question the usefulness of walking, suggesting that it is not strenuous enough to do any good. The value of walking depends on one's fitness level and personal exercise goals. Walking is an excellent activity for many people because just about anyone can do it, it can be done almost anywhere (in a park, at the mall, around your neighborhood), it's free, and you don't need any equipment other than a pair of shoes and socks. Walking is not only a good activity for most people, it is actually the first exercise you ever did. How old were you when you took your first step?

Notes

1. *proposed by Knuttgen.* Knuttgen, H. G. (2003). What is exercise? A primer for practitioners. *Physician and Sportsmedicine, 31,* 31-42.

2. *"spontaneous physical activity."* Donnelly, J. E., & Smith, B. K. (2005). Is exercise effective for weight loss with *ad libitum* diet? Energy balance, compensation, and gender differences. *Exercise and Sport Sciences Reviews, 33,* 169-174.

3. *Corbin and Lindsey's.* Corbin, C. B., & Lindsey, R. (1997). *Concepts of fitness and wellness with laboratories* (2nd ed.). Boston: WCB/McGraw-Hill.

4. *The National Athletic Trainers Association.* National Athletic Trainers Association (2003). Physical activity definition. Available: www.nata.org/about/activitydefinition.html.

5. *American College of Sports Medicine (ACSM).* American College of Sports Medicine, (1998). Position stand: The recommended quantity and quality of exercise for developing and maintaining cardiorespiratory and muscular fitness, and flexibility in healthy adults. *Medicine & Science in Sports and Exercise, 30,* 975-991.

6. *Lore of Running:* Noakes, T. (2003 updated 4th ed.). *Lore of Running.* Champaign, IL: Human Kinetics.

7. *Physical Fitness:* Retrieved from web, May 2007, from http://cyberparent.com/fitness/five.htm

8. *the exerciser's goals.* Knuttgen, H. G. (2003). What is Exercise: A Primer for Practitioners. *Physician and Sportsmedicine, 31,* 31-42.

9. *in TIME magazine.* Miranda, C. A., & Park, A. (June, 2005). Getting fit: The shape of a nation. *Time.* New York: Time, Inc.

10. *"Big Fat Lies."* Gaesser, G. A. (2002). *Big Fat Lies: The Truth about Your Weight and Your Health..* Carlsbad, CA: Gürze Books.

11. *Després and colleagues.* Després, J. P., Tremblay, A., Moorjani, S., Lupien, P. J., Theriault, G., Nadeau, A., & Bouchard, C. (1990). Long-term exercise training with constant energy intake: 3 effects on plasma lipoprotein levels. *International Journal of Obesity, 14,* 85-94.

12. *Després:* Després, J. P. (2002). The metabolic syndrome. In C. G. Fairburn & K. D. Brownell (Eds.), *Eating disorders and obesity: A comprehensive handbook* (2nd ed.), pp. 477-483. New York: The Guilford Press. .

13. *quality of life.* Corbin, C. B., & Lindsey, R. (1997). *Concepts of fitness and wellness with laboratories* (2nd ed.). Boston: WCB/McGraw-Hill.

14. *health but not fitness.* American College of Sports Medicine (1998). Position stand: The recommended quantity and quality of exercise for developing and maintaining cardiorespiratory and muscular fitness, and flexibility in healthy adults. *Medicine & Science in Sports and Exercise, 30,* 975-991.

15. *for men than women.* Donnelly, J. E., & Smith, B. K. (2005). Is exercise effective for weight loss with *ad libitum* diet: Energy balance, compensation, and gender differences. *Exercise and Sport Sciences Reviews, 33,* 169-174.

16. *high-carbohydrate foods.* Lowe MR: Self-regulation of energy intake in the prevention and treatment of obesity. Is it feasible? *Obes Res* 11:44S-59S, 2003.

17. *high-carbohydrate foods.* Berthoud HR: Neural systems controlling food intake and energy balance in the modern world. *Curr Opin Clin Nutr Metab Care* 6:615-620, 2003.

18. *energy availability.* Loucks, A. B. (2003). Energy availability, not body fatness, regulates reproductive function in women. *Exercise and Sports Sciences Review, 31,* 144-148.

19. *we recommend and Gaesser suggests.* Gaesser, G. A. (2002). *Big Fat Lies: The Truth about Your Weight and Your Health.* Carlsbad, CA: Gürze Books.

20. *MET system is available online.* Ainsworth, B. E. (2002, January). The compendium of physical activities tracking guide. Available: http://prevention.sph.sc.edu/tools/docs/documents_compendium.pdf .

21. Harris, JA,, & Benedict, FG. (1919). *A Biometric Study of Basal Metabolism in Man.* Washington DC, Carnegie Institute of Washington.

22. *"power" (rate of performing work).* Knuttgen, H. G. (2003). What is exercise? A primer for practitioners. *Physician and Sportsmedicine, 31,* 31-42.

23. *Self-Administered Physical Activity Checklist.* Sallis J.F., Strikmiller P.K., Harasha D.W., et al. (1996). Validation of interviewer and self-administered checklists for fifth grade students. *Medicine & Science in Sports and Exercise* 28:840-851.

24. *Minnesota Leisure Time Physical Activity Questionnaire.* Jacobs D.R. Jr., Ainsworth B.E., Hartman T.J., Leon A.S. (1993). A simultaneous evaluation of 10 commonly used physical activity questionnaires. *Medicine & Science in Sports and Exercise* 25:81-91.

25. *Scale for the Elderly:* Sallis, J. F. & Zabinski, M. F. (2002). Measurement of physical activity. In C. G. Fairburn & K. D. Brownell (Eds.), *Eating Disorders and Obesity: A Comprehensive Handbook* (2nd ed.), pp. 136-140. New York: The Guilford Press.

CHAPTER 3

Characteristics and Hazards of Overexercise

Excessive exercise can have serious physical and emotional consequences. Using qualitative and quantitative factors, in this chapter we define and describe how and why people overexercise and the consequences. We differentiate between such related terms as "obligatory" and "compulsive" exercise and also provide a questionnaire to help readers determine whether or not their workout routine is healthy or unhealthy.

In our society, exercise is viewed as a positive behavior, something that is a "good" thing to do. People who exercise regularly are thought of as healthy, motivated, and disciplined. They report feeling better, both physically and psychologically. But if some exercise is good, is a lot of exercise better? Can you get too much of this "good" thing? In essence, can exercise be "unhealthy?" Part of the answer to this question involves one's motivation. People exercise for many reasons: to improve their health, to have fun, to engage in competition, for social interaction, to lose or gain weight, or to "get in shape." To accomplish their goals, some people exercise more than others. But how much is too much?

Excessive Exercise: Quantity, Quality, Health and Balance

Determining whether or not an individual's exercise regimen is excessive can be a complicated process. We can simplify things if we begin with a practical and intuitive definition that includes both *quantitative* and *qualitative* factors. Exercise can be excessive in terms of: number or "how many" (50 vs. 500 sit-ups), frequency or "how often" (twice a week vs. more than once per day), duration or "how long" (a 20-minute session vs. so much time that it interferes with normal daily activities), or intensity or "how hard" (feel good vs. pain). Another way of determining whether or not a person is overexercising is to consider whether or not the amount and intensity is appropriate for that person's age group, circumstances, and/or health status. For example, a 15-year-old girl on the school volleyball team might practice 1–2 hours three times per week, compete one hour a week, and roller blade with her friends twice a week for two hours at a time. This is an appropriate amount of exercise for a healthy teenager. On the other hand, if she did all this plus ran for an hour every day and began to lose weight, her regimen would probably be excessive. Additionally, it would be even more inappropriate and unhealthy if she exercised while injured or if it interfered with everyday activities and relationships. It all depends on the individual and the circumstances.

Terms to Describe Excessive Exercise

Many terms are used to describe excessive exercise, including: compulsive, obligatory, addictive, dependence, and abuse. These describe the same basic set of behaviors and attitudes but with subtle differences. Some terms such as "compulsive" or "obligatory" suggest a connection to personality or motivational factors. However, just because someone is compulsive, doesn't mean that person is an overexerciser. Herein lies part of the difficulty.

Compulsive exercise means the individual engages in a variety of rituals, typically feeling compelled to exercise in the *same* way, at the *same* time, for the *same* duration, and the *same* exercises every day. While an urge to be active can be functional and healthy, someone who is compulsive often feels an overwhelming push or drive to exercise that may indicate negative emotional states, such as fear, guilt, or anxiety. Exercising temporarily eases these feelings. Many compulsive exercisers are unaware of this connection. The person may not actually be overdoing it physically, but the exercise may be unbalanced because of the compulsive way in which it is used to cope with negative feelings that could be managed in healthier ways.

> Compulsive exercise means a person feels compelled to exercise a certain way or at a certain time.

Obligatory exercise means the individual *must* exercise. For this type of person, *not* exercising is simply *not* an option. The obligatory exerciser will workout despite circumstances that would preclude exercise for most other people, including when that person is ill or injured. If also compulsive, the individual may follow the same exercise routine for years without missing a single day. The fact that someone admits to or feels proud of this type of behavior suggests that he or she sees nothing wrong with it, that it should be viewed as an accomplishment. The person may also continue his regimen to maintain a record of consecutive days, months, or years. Unfortunately, various specialty magazines, such as *Runner's World*, praise this type of behavior. Clearly, the obligatory exerciser would disagree with our recommendation to rest at least one day per week, which is in keeping with many sports medicine groups such as the American College of Sports Medicine[1] and governing bodies such

> Obligatory exercise means the person must exercise no matter what the circumstances.

as the National Collegiate Athletic Association (NCAA).[2] For instance, the NCAA limits what a coach can require from an athlete to 20 hours per week.

The relationship between compulsive and obligatory exercise can become rather complex. Some excessive exercisers are compulsive, some are obligatory, and some are both. Interestingly, a few people exercise in ways that have both obligatory and compulsive aspects, but their exercise is not excessive. Let's take a look at Steve.

Steve has to run first thing every day and will adjust his schedule as necessary. His running is obligatory but is less compulsive in that he can make adjustments when life events dictate. For example, he is just as comfortable running at 4 o'clock as he is at 6 o'clock. Also, if he is in a location that is not conducive to running, he runs in place instead. However, he does not run excessive mileage, duration, or intensity. In fact, over the years, he has run less mileage, less duration, and at a slower speed. Steve also likes to lift weights, but his lifting is not excessive, compulsive, or obligatory. When his schedule allows, he likes to lift daily. He does not lift excessive weight, do excessive repetitions or sets, nor does he lift for a long period of time. He is even more adaptive with his lifting than his running. For example, if he is traveling and does not have the availability of a gym, he can forego lifting for a week or more without any negative effects (e.g., anxiety). Although there are some compulsive and obligatory aspects to his exercise regimen, Steve's routine is generally healthy and not excessive.

Additional terms sometimes used in relation to excessive, compulsive, and obligatory exercise include the closely-related *exercise dependence* and *exercise addiction*. "Dependence" and "addiction" are usually associated with behaviors that are viewed as having negative health and lifestyle consequences and which are out of a person's control, such as addiction to alcohol or drugs. The reasons for *exercise addiction* often focus on levels of brain chemicals such as endorphins or neurotransmitters, like serotonin and dopamine. These are natural substances that are known to produce a sense of euphoria during and/or after exercise. However, some experts suggest that the "high" associated with exercise is also psychological in nature. While various authors say that exercise addiction can be positive, we believe that a behavior is not necessarily positive or negative when viewed alone. Rather, the context in which the exercise occurs determines whether it has a beneficial or toxic effect on a person's health and life.

The final term that we address is *exercise abuse,*[3] which incorporates many of the previously mentioned definitions. There are three key signs:

1. Reliance on physical activity as the primary means of coping with stress

2. Exercise continued even when ill or injured

3. Withdrawal symptoms (insomnia, change in appetite, trouble concentrating, moodiness, etc.) if exercise is reduced or stopped

Regardless of which term is used, excessive exercise is often related to an individual's personality, attitudes, and emotions—in essence, from the psychological part of the person. In that regard, what do psychiatry and psychology have to say about excessive exercise? The *Diagnostic and Statistical Manual of Mental Disorders*[4] defines exercise as excessive "when it significantly interferes with important activities, when it occurs at inappropriate times or in inappropriate settings, or when the individual continues to exercise despite injury or other medical complications" (p.546).

Activity Anorexia

Overexercise has been studied using animals. This research was initiated in part to understand why many individuals suffering from anorexia nervosa also engage in excessive exercise. The *activity anorexia* model describes the process that allegedly precipitates or triggers anorexia nervosa in many individuals.[5] Conventional wisdom tells us that burning calories should result in hunger, or a need to eat, in order to replace the fuel that has been burned. However, at least one animal model suggests the converse. That is, some animals experience a decreased appetite the more they exercise. Studies indicate that these animals can quite literally exercise themselves to death.

> Leptin is a protein hormone that helps regulate weight, metabolism, and energy expenditure.

Some researchers suggest that the preceding animal model can explain activity anorexia in many humans. In our own clinical practice, we have certainly worked with anorexic patients who appear to engage in a process that is consistent with activity anorexia. Several theories attempt to explain this unusual phenomenon, which typically involve certain neurobiological processes that interact to inhibit eating in exercising individuals. One of the more recent theories involves *leptin*, a protein hormone that helps regulate weight, metabolism, and energy expenditure. A low leptin level, caused by food restriction, may trigger the same increased activity levels in anorexic patients as is observed in food-deprived animals. This process is referred to as *semi-starvation-induced hyperactivity.*[6]

An interesting side note that lends credence to neurobiological theories involves long-distance runners, many of whom report that they have no appetite during and after running, especially if it is heavy and prolonged—like the conditions of a marathon. As mentioned previously, some of our anorexic patients also seem to experience decreased appetite following exercise. Perhaps the most illustrative is Claire.

Claire's eating disorder began after a period of unhealthy dieting combined with what became overexercise. She claimed that exercising made her feel less tense or anxious. Regrettably, this relaxed state did not last long. She soon felt the need to exercise again or else would become even more tense. Claire believed that exercise was the only thing that would make her feel better. Her situation was further complicated in that she felt no need or desire to eat. In fact, she reported that the more she exercised, the less she wanted to eat. Obviously, her behavior resulted in a negative energy balance and weight loss.

Although Claire maintained that she was not exercising to lose weight and only to feel better, she was placed on exercise restriction. Yet her drive was so strong that she secretly exercised against treatment advice and experienced dangerous weight loss. Eventually, with the help of psychotherapy, she was finally able to find other ways to manage her anxiety.

Physical Consequences of Overexercise

Many problems can occur with excessive exercise, from minor aches and pains to serious complications that could endanger your life.

Sex hormone levels can decrease to the point that the reproductive system may be negatively affected. A complete shutdown of the menstrual cycle is common in women who overexercise, especially for those who also have low body weight. The situation for men is less clear, but it is known that excessive exercise in men can lead to decreased testosterone levels. However, research results on how this affects sperm quantity, quality, and movement are currently inconclusive.

Bone health is related to sex hormones and exercise. When functioning properly, the human body is simultaneously building up and breaking down bone, which is a delicate balance. Without sex hormones (estrogen in women, testosterone in men), the human body cannot build bone mass, but does continue to break it down, which can cause bones to become thin, weak, and brittle, resulting in an increased risk for fractures, especially stress fractures. The American Academy of Orthopedic Surgeons defines a *stress fracture*[7] as an overuse injury that occurs when the muscles are fatigued and unable to absorb added shock. The fatigued muscle transfers the overload of stress to the bone causing a tiny crack called a "stress fracture." Decreased bone density (defined as osteopenia or osteoporosis depending on the severity of bone loss) increases vulnerability to stress fractures. Figure 3.1 is an illustration of a stress fracture of the metatarsal bone in the foot. Ironically, weight-bearing exercise is necessary for bone growth, but too much can actually decrease hormone levels, resulting in bone loss.

FIGURE 3.1. Stress Fracture of Metatarsal Bone

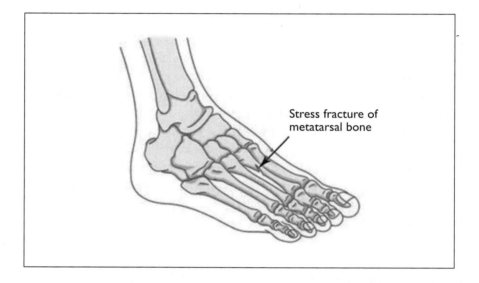

Stress fracture of metatarsal bone

Stress fractures are overuse injuries that occur when the muscles are fatigued and unable to absorb added shock. The fatigued muscle transfers the overload of stress to the bone causing a tiny crack which is called a stress fracture.

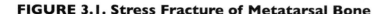

Some people suffer *musculoskeletal*—or structure and movement—problems from doing too much when it would be healthier to take a break. For instance, running on a sprained ankle is not a good idea and can lead to further bodily damage. Some people develop overuse injuries, which usually involve muscles or bones and joints. When an individual feels pain, the body is literally communicating that something is wrong. If the symptom is ignored, it tends to worsen. Individuals who experience overuse injuries usually ignore, deny, or mislabel their body signals. Whatever the cause of the stress fracture, when that activity is continued, the damage gets worse. These are the people who "talk at" rather than "listen to" their bodies and voice clichés such as "no pain, no gain" or "pain is simply weakness leaving the body." They may even tell themselves to "run through the pain," a sure warning sign that something is wrong.

Although regular, moderate exercise is reported to have a positive effect on the body's immunity, intense exercise for extended periods of time may actually cause *decreased immune function* in some individuals,[8] which puts the body at a greater risk of infection. Researchers suggest that this lowered immunity is probably related to stress hormones (i.e., cortisol and adrenaline) that are released during intense endurance exercise.

Dangers of excessive exercise also include potentially fatal complications that involve the cardiovascular system, such as *Sudden Arrhythmia Death Syndrome.*[9] By definition, this is a death that occurs within one hour of the onset of symptoms in a person without a previously recognized heart problem. Over 90% of victims who die have a pre-existing cardiac abnormality that was not diagnosed. In 2004, the International Olympic Committee adopted the Lausanne Recommendations for "Sudden Cardiovascular Death in Sport," a pre-participation cardiovascular screening for elite athletes under 35 years. The steps include obtaining a personal history to assess possible symptoms of heart disease, a family history to detect possible genetic risk for early heart disease, a physical examination targeting specific signs suggestive of heart disease, and a 12-lead resting electrocardiogram after the onset of puberty. Use Table 3.1 to detect underlying symptoms of hidden heart disease and Table 3.2 to determine if you have a genetic risk.

TABLE 3.1. Personal History Suggesting Heart Problems

Directions: If you answer yes to one or more of the following questions you should consult with your doctor before beginning or continuing a vigorous or competitive exercise routine.

Personal history: Questionnaire by examining physician	YES	NO
Have you ever fainted or passed out when exercising?		
Do you ever have chest tightness?		
Does running ever cause chest tightness?		
Have you ever had chest tightness, cough, or wheezing which made it difficult for you to perform in sports?		
Have you ever been treated/hospitalized for asthma?		
Have you ever had a seizure?		

Continued on next page

Personal history: Questionnaire by examining physician (Continued)	YES	NO
Have you ever been told that you have epilepsy?		
Have you ever been told to give up sports because of health problems?		
Have you ever been told you have high blood pressure?		
Have you ever been told you have high cholesterol?		
Do you have trouble breathing or do you cough during or after activity?		
Have you ever been dizzy during or after exercise?		
Have you ever had chest pain during or after exercise?		
Do you have or have you ever had racing of your heart or skipped heartbeats?		
Do you get tired more quickly than your friends do during exercise?		
Have you ever been told you have a heart murmur?		
Have you ever been told you have a heart arrhythmia?		
Do you have any other history of heart problems?		
Have you had a severe viral infection (for example myocarditis or mononucleosis) within the last month?		
Have you ever been told you have rheumatic fever?		
Do you have any allergies?		
Are you taking any medications at the present time?		
Have you routinely taken any medication in the past two years?		

From "Sudden Cardiovascular Death in Sport: Lausanne Recommendations." Under the umbrella IOC Medical Commission, 10 December 2004. Adapted and used with permission.

TABLE 3.2. Family History Suggestive of Heart Disease

Directions: If you answer yes to one or more of the following questions you should consult with your doctor before beginning or continuing a vigorous or competitive exercise routine.

Family history: Questionnaire by examining physician	YES	NO
Has anyone in your family less than 50 years old:		
Died suddenly and unexpectedly?		
Been treated for recurrent fainting?		
Had unexplained seizure problems?		
Had unexplained drowning while swimming?		
Had an unexplained car accident?		
Had heart transplantation?		
Had a pacemaker or defibrillator implanted?		
Been treated for irregular heart beat?		
Had heart surgery?		
Has anyone in your family experienced sudden infant death?		
Has anyone in your family been told they have Marfan syndrome?		

From "Sudden Cardiovascular Death in Sport: Lausanne Recommendations." Under the umbrella IOC Medical Commission, 10 December 2004. Adapted and used with permission.

Some individuals have a *prolonged QT interval,* which is a potentially fatal abnormality in the rhythm of the heart. This could lead to ventricular arrhythmias and sudden death. This condition can be detected by an electrocardiogram. If you have a family history of cardiac problems or if you have even minor symptoms that might indicate heart disease, such as shortness of breath or chest pain, a consultation with a primary care physician prior to undertaking an exercise program is advised. Your doctor may request an electro-cardiogram to assess your QT interval or other rhythm abnormalities. Asking your doctor about a reasonable and safe exercise program *before* you begin is especially important if you are diagnosed with a prolonged QT interval.

FIGURE 3.2. QT Interval Prolongation

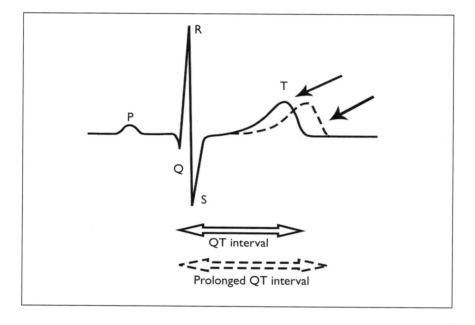

The QT interval can be prolonged for many reasons, including genetic vulnerability, underlying heart disease, or many different medicines. Exercising with a prolonged QT interval can be deadly. Adapted from Abriel H, Schlapfer J, Keller DJ, et al: Molecular and clinical determinants of drug-induced long QT syndrome: an iatrogenic channelopathy. *Swiss Medical Weekly* 27: 685-694, 2004. Used with permission.

During exercise, maintaining normal fluid (water) and electrolyte levels is crucial. Electrolytes include sodium and chloride, which are the components of salt. Sweat includes water and salt, so it is important to replenish these to avoid *dehydration* and *heat stroke* from high sweat rates. But, overhydration from drinking more fluid than is lost from sweat can also be dangerous and is the leading cause of exercise-induced *hyponatremia* (which is a sodium level that is too low). Hyponatremia can result in brain problems (with initial symptoms of confusion and disorientation) and lung problems (with an initial symptom of shortness of breath) and even death. Determining and maintaining normal hydration and sodium levels in elite athletes or intense exercisers is beyond the scope of this book, but the 2007 Position Stand on Exercise and Fluid Replacement[10] by the American College of Sports Medicine is very informative and can be found online.

TABLE 3.3. Working Heart Range Calculation

Both men and women can use the following formulas to find the lower and upper heart rates for moderate and vigorous physical activity for your age. Stay within this range while exercising for a beneficial cardiovascular workout.

Moderate Intensity Physical Activity (50–70% maximum heart rate)

lower heart rate = (220 – your age) x 0.50 = heartbeats per minute
upper heart rate = (220 – your age) x 0.70 = heartbeats per minute
range for moderate physical activity = lower–upper heartbeats per minute

Example: The calculations for a 45-year-old are as follows.
lower heart rate = (220 – 45 years) x 0.50 = 88 heartbeats per minute
upper heart rate = (220 – 45 years) x 0.70 = 123 heartbeats per minute
range for moderate physical activity = 88–123 heartbeats per minute

Vigorous Intensity Physical Activity (70–85% maximum heart rate)

lower heart rate = (220 – your age) x 0.70 = heartbeats per minute
upper heart rate = (220 – your age) x 0.85 = heartbeats per minute
range for vigorous physical activity = lower–upper heartbeats per minute

Example: The calculations for a 45-year-old are as follows.
lower heart rate = (220 – 45 years) x 0.70 = 123 heartbeats per minute
upper heart rate = (220 – 45 years) x 0.85 = 149 heartbeats per minute
range for vigorous physical activity = 123–149 heartbeats per minute

Monitoring your heart rate during and soon after exercise to remain in a safe range can also be important. Several ways of estimating this range are available. As shown in Table 3.3, if you are a 45-year-old man or woman and in good health, your working heart range for moderately intense physical activity is between 88–123 heartbeats per minute (or 14–20 heartbeats per 10 seconds). Immediately *stop* exercising if you experience symptoms such as muscle cramps, light-headedness, chest pain, sudden fatigue, profuse sweating, confusion, disorientation, or sudden shortness of breath. These symptoms can be indications of very serious complications and should be evaluated promptly by a health care professional. Some of these symptoms (for example, light-headedness or chest pain) *may* be due to dehydration and some (for example confusion or disorientation) *may* be due to hyponatremia, but this is not always easy to determine yourself. Do not begin exercising again until the symptoms have completely resolved. Also, determine if you were overhydrated or underhydrated, and work toward achieving normal hydration—a healthy balance of fluid and electrolytes.

There may be more warning signs of potential problems among adults who engage in unhealthy exercise than among normal-weight adolescents, who are usually considered to be in good health. For adults who visit their doctor on a regular basis, certain risk factors (e.g., hypertension or obesity) may be routinely identified; however, note that the possibility of heart abnormalities is often overlooked in underweight adults, especially women. Moreover, men are often lax about visiting their primary care physician for regular check-ups and frequently do not seek advice before starting an exercise program. They may be jeopardizing their health due to undetected risk factors.

Psychological Aspects of Overexercise

We have already alluded to many of the ways that overexercise can affect mental and emotional health. It can add considerable stress and strain when responsibilities and relationships are subordinated to working out. If you rely on unhealthy exercise to cope with life's issues, you may become depressed, anxious, irritable, or uneasy when you skip it. Such overexercisers will sometimes rationalize that they are exercising for their health, while actually they may be putting their health at risk. Interestingly, men are more apt to use health as a rationale than women, who are more inclined to use weight control.

Also, many people who exercise excessively do so alone, because they feel others will interfere with the length or intensity of their routine. Although this is not to say that everyone who exercises alone does so in an unhealthy manner. For some, this solitary activity is a way to avoid people and may be taking away from potentially satisfying social opportunities.

Even competitive athletes—a group often considered to be "healthy"—can suffer psychological problems. Research suggests that athletes who train too much and experience the "overtraining syndrome"[11] can suffer from a negative shift in mood (depression).[12] We will discuss this more in the next chapter.

For some individuals, exercise becomes part of an unhealthy relationship with eating and weight. It can be used to compensate for, or legitimize, eating. Or, it can be used to maintain an unhealthy negative energy balance. If you intentionally eat less when you are unable to exercise, especially when you are hungry, you have a problem. A prime example of such behavior is the following patient.

A Patient Example

Kiko is a 35-year-old woman who developed anorexia nervosa when she was 21. She initially lost weight by restricting her food intake and then began exercising to lose even more. If Kiko didn't exercise, she wouldn't eat because she felt she didn't deserve food. She entered treatment to work on her eating disorder, poor body image, and low self-esteem, and gradually gained back some weight. Unfortunately, she then developed a pattern in which she had to exercise in order to allow herself to eat, increasing her exercise from one to eventually six hours per day. She began to dread mornings because she was tired yet felt compelled to complete her program. She became unable to work and her parents had to provide financial support. Ultimately, she broke her ankle while running and had to stop altogether. During this time she became profoundly depressed and had to be hospitalized for more intense treatment.

Am I Overexercising?

The first step in determining whether or not you are exercising too much is to take an honest and objective look at your life. Ask yourself if your routine negatively impacts your physical, emotional, or psychological health. Does it interfere with everyday activities such as school, work, or relationships? If so, you are probably overexercising and need to modify your regimen as well as your attitude. As was suggested previously, other indicators include exercise that occurs at inappropriate times or settings or continues despite injury or other medical complications.[13] For example, if you absolutely must exercise even if your children need your attention, then your routine is inappropriate. If you have an injured knee and your doctor advises you not to run until it heals but you continue to run anyway, you are being driven by unhealthy psychological forces.

The relevant issue here is not how much one exercises but the *appropriateness* of the given situation.

Another way to think about overexercise is within the framework of *energy balance*, which occurs when the calories consumed equal the energy expended. With so much emphasis on the health problems associated with being overweight or obese, we sometimes forget that being undernourished or underweight is also unhealthy. Many people mistakenly believe that a person can neither be too thin nor have a body-fat ratio that is too low. In reality, this is *not* the case. An example of imbalance would be the use of physical activity to achieve an *energy deficit* that results in weight loss. Sometimes this is appropriate behavior—a temporary and slight increase in exercise or a reduction in calorie intake is acceptable if one needs to lose weight for health purposes. On the other hand, if an individual is at a normal or low weight and has a normal body composition, an energy deficit is inappropriate.

Of course there are exceptions. One example would be a recruit in boot camp who needs to increase muscle mass over fat mass. Another example might be an elite athlete in training who needs a sport-specific body size and/or composition and mix of energy stores. Yet another might be a person suffering from osteoarthritis or stiff joints. In this case, a slight increase in muscle mass combined with a slightly lower-than-normal body weight might help increase one's mobility, as long as she is being carefully monitored by her health care practitioners.

Questionnaires to Assess Exercise

Several researchers have tried to devise questionnaires or scales that will help you or your doctor determine if you are abusing exercise. The Obligatory Exercise Questionnaire[14] is shown in Table 3.4. You are encouraged to take this test to evaluate your particular situation. The test takes about 5 minutes to complete. The higher the score, the more likely it is that exercise may be excessive. If the score suggests that exercise is a problem, it is important to make an appointment to talk to your doctor and/or counselor.

TABLE 3.4. The Obligatory Exercise Questionnaire

By J.K. Thompson and L. Pasman

Directions: Listed below is a series of statements about people's exercise habits. Please circle the number that reflects how often you make the following statements:

I – NEVER   2 – SOMETIMES   3 – USUALLY   4 – ALWAYS

1. I engage in physical exercise on a daily basis.   1   2   3   4

2. I engage in one/more of the following forms of exercise: walking, jogging/running or weight lifting.   1   2   3   4

3. I exercise more than three days per week.   1   2   3   4

4. When I don't exercise I feel guilty.   1   2   3   4

5. I sometimes feel like I don't want to exercise, but I go ahead and push myself anyway.   1   2   3   4

6. My best friend likes to exercise.   1   2   3   4

7. When I miss an exercise session, I feel concerned about my body possibly getting out of shape.   1   2   3   4

8. If I have planned to exercise at a particular time and something unexpected comes up (like an old friend comes to visit or I have some work to do that needs immediate attention) I will usually skip my exercise for that day.   1   2   3   4

9. If I miss a planned workout, I attempt to make up for it the next day.   1   2   3   4

10. I may miss a day of exercise for no good reason.   1   2   3   4

11. Sometimes, I feel a need to exercise twice in one day, even though I may feel a little tired.   1   2   3   4

12. If I feel I have overeaten, I will try to make up for it by increasing the amount I exercise.   1   2   3   4

13. When I miss a scheduled exercise session I may feel tense, irritable or depressed.   1   2   3   4

Contiued on next page

14. Sometimes, I find that my mind wanders to thoughts about exercising.   1 2 3 4

15. I have had daydreams about exercising.   1 2 3 4

16. I keep a record of my exercise performance, such as how long I work out, how far or fast I run.   1 2 3 4

17. I have experienced a feeling of euphoria or a "high" during or after an exercise session.   1 2 3 4

18. I frequently "push myself to the limits."   1 2 3 4

19. I have exercised when advised against such activity (i.e., by a doctor, friend, etc.).   1 2 3 4

20. I will engage in other forms of exercise if I am unable to engage in my usual form of exercise.   1 2 3 4

Scoring: To score the questionnaire, first reverse the scores for items 8 and 10 (for example, if you wrote "always 4" for Item #8, then reverse it to "1") and then obtain the total. If you score 30 or less, your exercise is probably not obligatory. Scores between 30 and 40 indicate there is reason for mild concern. Scores between 40 and 50 suggest you may have moderate problems with obligatory exercise. Scores above 50 mean you should consider finding ways to moderate your exercise. This questionnaire was used with permission.

At Risk for Excessive Exercise: Individuals with Eating Disorders

Increased levels of activity have been described among patients with anorexia nervosa for over 100 years. Sir William Gull, one of the first physicians to describe this illness wrote, "For it seemed hardly possible that a body so wasted could undergo the exercise which seemed agreeable."[15] This type of overactivity has been observed in both people with anorexia nervosa and bulimia nervosa and has been described in a variety of ways, including hyperactivity, motor restlessness, excessive exercise, and high level exercise. Just as it is not easy to determine how healthy or balanced exercise is in the general population, it is especially difficult to recognize overexercise among people with eating disorders.

In one study, about half of female patients with either anorexia nervosa or bulimia nervosa were regarded as exercising too much prior to hospitalization for their eating disorder.[16] Not surprisingly, many of these individuals were more active than others their age when they were young. About the same percentage (50%) of women say that regular exercise preceded dieting during the development of their illness. Most patients say that as their illness worsened their physical activity progressed from a voluntary and usually enjoyable endeavor to an obsessive or out-of-control activity that they could not stop.

Estimates of the prevalence of excessive exercise among eating disorder patients range from 33% to over 80%.[17] Patients who overexercise are more likely to have other, more severe eating-disorder symptoms, including greater body dissatisfaction, more preoccupation with weight, and a greater drive for thinness than do eating disorder patients who maintain low levels of exercise. Excessive activity or hyperactivity is one of the last symptoms to improve with treatment, and patients who overexercise often need a longer period for recovery.[18] The excessive commitment to exercise and dietary restraint experienced by so many people with anorexia nervosa may be partially explained by their perfectionism. Also, those who continue to exercise compulsively after they are discharged from a treatment center are more likely to have a poor outcome than those with moderate exercise levels,[19] whereas people who learned to adjust, rather than suppress, exercise during recovery from an eating disorder had a better long-term outcome.[20]

> Moderation, flexibility, and balance are key to appropriate exercise.

Many treatment programs use access to exercise as a reward for weight gain. We believe it is more appropriate to define moderate exercise as a goal, not a reward, because a complete lack of exercise is also unhealthy. Our position is that moderation, flexibility, and balance applied to exercise are likely to result in better health.

Notes

1. *American College of Sports Medicine.* American College of Sports Medicine. (1998). Position stand: The recommended quantity and quality of exercise for developing and maintaining cardio-respiratory and muscular fitness, and flexibility in healthy adults. *Medicine and Science in Sports and Exercise, 30,* 975-991.

2. *National Collegiate Athletic Association.* National Collegiate Athletic Association (2003). 2002-2003 *NCAA division I manual.* Indianapolis, IN: The National Collegiate Athletic Association.

3. *address is exercise abuse.* Raglin, J. S., & Moger, L. (1999). Adverse consequences of physical activity: When more is too much. In J. M. Rippe (Ed.), *Lifestyle Medicine* (pp. 998-1004), Malden, MA: Blackwell Science.

4. *Diagnostic and Statistical Manual of Mental Disorders.* American Psychiatric Association. (1994). *Diagnostic and Statistical Manual of Mental Disorders* (4ᵗʰ ed.). Washington, DC: Author.

5. *anorexia nervosa in many individuals.* Epling, W. F., & Pierce, W. D. (1996). *Activity anorexia: Theory, research, and treatment.* Mahwah, NJ: Lawrence Erlbaum Associates, Inc.

6. *semi-starvation-induced hyperactivity.* Hebebrand, J., Exner, C., Hebebrand, K., Holtkamp, C., Casper, R. C., Remschmidt, H., Herpertz-Dalhmann, B, Klingenspor, M. (2003). Hyperactivity in patients with anorexia nervosa and in semistarved rats: Evidence for a pivotal role of hypoleptinemia. *Physiology and Behavior, 79,* 25-37.

7. *defines a stress fracture.* American Academy of Orthopedic Surgeons. Available: http://orthoinfo.org/fact/thr_report.cfm?thread_id=46.

8. *immune function in some individuals.* Nieman, D. C.(2003). Current perspective on exercise immunology. *Current Sports Medicine Reports, 2,* 239-242.

9. *Sudden Arrhythmia Death Syndrome.* Meyer JS, Mehdirad A, Salem BI, Kulikowski A, Kalikowski P (2003). Sudden arrhythmia death syndrome: importance of the long QT syndrome. *American Family Physician,* 68, 483-488.

10. *Exercise and Fluid Replacement.* American College of Sports Medicine Position Stand (2007). Available: http://www.acsm-msse.org.

11. *overtraining syndrome.* Raglin, J.D., & Wilson, G.S. (2000). *Overtraining in athletes.* In Y.L. Hanin (Ed.), *Emotions in Sport* (pp. 191-207). Champaign, IL: Human Kinetics.

12. *shift in mood (depression).* Raglin, J.D., & Wilson, G.S. (2000). *Overtraining in athletes.* In Y.L. Hanin (Ed.), *Emotions in Sport* (pp. 191-207). Champaign, IL: Human Kinetics.

13. *or other medical complications.* American Psychiatric Association. (1994). *Diagnostic and Statistical Manual of Mental Disorders* (4ᵗʰ ed.). Washington, DC: American Psychiatric Press.

14. *Obligatory Exercise Questionnaire.* Pasman, L. J., & Thompson, J. K. (1988). Body image and eating disturbance in obligatory runners, obligatory weightlifters, and sedentary individuals. *International Journal of Eating Disorders, 7,* 759-769.

15. *exercise which seemed agreeable:* Gull, W. W. (1874). Anorexia nervosa (apepsia hysterica, anorexia hysterica). *Translations of the Clinical Society of London, 7,* 22-28.

16. *hospitalization for their eating disorder.* Solenberger, S. E. (2001). Exercise and eating disorders: A 3-year inpatient hospital record analysis. *Eating Behaviors, 2,* 151-168.

17. *from 33% to more than 80%.* Katz, J. L., (1996). Clinical observations on the physical activity of anorexia nervosa. In W. F. Epling & W. D. Pierce (Eds.), *Activity Anorexia: Theory, Research, and Treatment* (pp. 199-207). Mahwah, NJ: Lawrence Erlbaum Associates, Inc.

18. *longer period for recovery.* Solenberger, S. E. (2001). Exercise and Eating Disorders: A 3-year inpatient hospital record analysis. *Eating Behaviors, 2,* 151-168.

19. *with moderate exercise levels.* Strober, M., Freeman, R., & Morrell, W. (1997). The long-term course of severe anorexia nervosa in adolescents: Survival analysis of recovery, relapse, and outcome predictors over 10-15 years of a prospective study. *International Journal of Eating Disorders, 22,* 339-360.

20. *had a better long-term outcome.* Calogero, R. M., & Pedrotty, K. N. The practice and process of healthy exercise: Testing the effects of treating exercise abuse in women with eating disorders. *Eating Disorders: The Journal of Treatment and Prevention, 12:4,* 273-291

CHAPTER 4

Special Considerations for Competitive Athletes

In this chapter, we discuss exercise issues as they relate to "competitive" athletes, who are competing in sanctioned sports at all levels of competition. We describe the risks of complications some encounter, including the Female Athlete Triad, the overtraining syndrome ("staleness"), and mood disturbances. The special case of ultra-endurance athletes is discussed and our recommendation for balance in exercise is emphasized. Treatment recommendations for competitive athletes who develop problems are outlined; and finally, the erroneous belief in the sport world that weight loss or a decrease in body fat *invariably* improves performance is reviewed.

Many contemporary athletes would agree that improvements in their personal sport performance are related not only to the superior methods of modern training, but also to the stepped-up levels, which have increased significantly in recent years.[1] Unfortunately, this has caused more and more competitors to be at risk for excessive exercise. As difficult as it is to determine when exercise is unhealthy or unbalanced in the general public, it is even more difficult in competitive athletes. Although the amount of time an athlete can spend training is regulated by sport-governing bodies, such as the National Collegiate Athletic Association (NCAA), the belief that intense training produces positive results makes it difficult to recognize when an athlete might be doing too much, too often. Even though athletes are by definition more active than their non-athlete counterparts, a balance is still needed.

Is Intense Training an Attribute or a Symptom?

The difficulty with identifying unhealthy exercise in athletes involves distinguishing between the traits of a "good athlete" and the symptoms of an eating disorder. Characteristics found in competitors, such as perfectionism and an over-compliance to do whatever it takes to please others (especially coaches), are often the same as those found in individuals with anorexia nervosa.[2] Thus, it may be difficult to tell if an athlete is just working very hard or actually has a problem.

While unhealthy exercise is a common symptom for eating-disorder patients, especially those with anorexia nervosa, it is often overlooked or considered valuable in a sports environment. So, when an athlete trains harder and longer than her teammates, and she and her coach may believe she is simply doing it to enhance her performance, she may actually be engaged in pathological behavior indicative of a serious disorder. We are not saying that all hard-working athletes automatically have an eating disorder, but sometimes it is difficult to determine whether or not an individual is a good athlete, has anorexia nervosa, or both. Table 4.1 lists some of the similarities between the "good athlete" and the anorexic individual. If you exhibit any sign of unhealthy exercise or an eating disorder, we strongly encourage evaluation by a qualified healthcare professional.

> Many athletes exhibit signs of both unhealthy exercise and eating disorders.

TABLE 4.1. Similarities Between "Good Athlete" Traits and Anorexic Characteristics

"Good Athlete"	Anorexic Individual
Mental toughness	Asceticism
Commitment to training	Excessive exercise
Pursuit of excellence	Perfectionism
Coachability	Over-compliance
Unselfishness	Selflessness
Performance despite pain	Denial of discomfort

Thompson R.A, & Sherman, R.T. (1999). "Good athlete" traits and characteristics of anorexia nervosa. Are they similar? *Eating Disorders: The Journal of Treatment and Prevention, 7,* 181-190. Used with permission.

Female Athlete Triad

Women who train excessively are at risk for the *Female Athlete Triad*,[3] which includes symptoms of *disordered eating* (from simple dieting to clinical eating disorders), *amenorrhea* (absence of menstruation), and *osteoporosis* (loss of bone density). The Triad often begins with disordered eating, usually involving dietary restriction, coupled with too much exercise, resulting in low energy availability[4] (dietary intake minus exercise expenditure). When this imbalance occurs, especially if it is severe and persistent, the reproductive system can shut down to conserve energy, causing inadequate estrogen levels and amenorrhea. This, in turn, can result in osteoporosis, because bone growth and development require estrogen.

Although the Triad can affect female athletes at all levels of competition, physically active girls and young women who are not competitive athletes also appear to be at risk. A recent study found that 4.3% of elite athletes and 3.4% of non-athletes exhibited all three symptoms of the Triad, and the prevalence for those with only two symptoms ranges from 5.4% to 26.9% of elite athletes and 12.4% to 15.2% of non-athletes.[5] Although amenorrhea in athletes is often assumed to be due to low body weight or fat level, recent research suggests that it can also result from low energy availability.[6] In this case, a woman consumes insufficient calories to adequately fuel not only her physical activity but also the normal bodily processes related to health, growth, and development. Sometimes this insufficient intake is unintentional. Then again, in many cases, it is a willful attempt on the athlete's part to lose weight or body fat, either to meet an aesthetic standard of leanness and/or thinness for sports that are judged visually, or an attempt to enhance athletic performance.

> The Female Athlete Triad includes symptoms of disordered eating, amenorrhea, and osteoporosis.

Regarding the latter, a prevailing notion in the sports world is that a reduction in weight or body fat can improve athletic performance. There are flaws with that idea, which we discuss later in this chapter. Regardless, for most athletes, getting lean involves a combination of restricted eating (dieting) and increased training (exercise)—the two factors that contribute to insufficient energy availability. Thus, the erroneous belief that losing weight or body fat enhances athletic performance gives the athlete another rationale for training (exercising) more, but it also increases her risk for the Triad.

As previously stated, amenorrhea, if left untreated, can eventually lead to bone loss, first in the form of *osteopenia* (moderately low bone density) and eventually *osteoporosis* (very low bone density). A T-score is a measurement of bone density compared to what is normally expected in a healthy young female. According to diagnostic guidelines recommended by the World Health Organization, having a T-score between 1.0 and 2.5 standard deviations lower than the norm indicates osteopenia, and scores lower than 2.5 indicate osteoporosis. Treatment involves increasing caloric intake and/or de-creasing physical activity until normal menstruation returns, which may protect bone. A common misconception is that prescribing birth control pills (which may replace estrogen and result in withdrawl bleeding) will solve the problem. Menstrual bleeding is only a part of the normal menstrual cycle, and estrogen is only one of many factors that maintain normal bone mass. More information regarding the Female Athlete Triad is available by reading the International Olympic Committee Medical Commission's Position Stand[7] on the Internet.

Our discussion of the Female Athlete Triad should not give male athletes a false sense of security, because a similar phenomenon appears to occur in some men. As we mentioned in the previous chapter, research suggests that too much exercise may result in lowered levels of testosterone, which may increase the risk of bone density loss in a manner similar to lowered estrogen levels in women. Research also suggests that this may be due to what has been termed a *volume threshold* of training.[8] That is, up to a point, weight-bearing exercise helps build bone mass when adequate levels of calcium, Vitamin D, and testosterone are maintained. However, excessive levels may actually cause bone mass to break down. Although it is sometimes considered an "old woman's disease," according to the National Osteoporosis Foundation (NOF)[9], 2 million men in the U.S. have osteoporosis, while another 12 million are believed to be at risk. The true percentage may actually be higher because males and their physicians may not suspect or even consider it. The NOF reports that osteoporosis is overlooked in men and lists undiagnosed low levels of testosterone as a risk factor. The risk increases with age and there is also a dramatic increase in risk in men or boys with anorexia nervosa. Interestingly, recent research indicates that male anorexic patients suffer bone loss more often than their female counterparts, and the extent of bone loss is greater[10].

It is important to note that osteoporosis leads to an increased likelihood of fractures, especially stress fractures, and unhealthy exercise can result in joint injuries, often to the knee. Women are particularly prone to knee damage (especially the anterior cruciate ligament) when compared to men.

FIGURE 4.1. Anterior Cruciate Ligament of the Knee

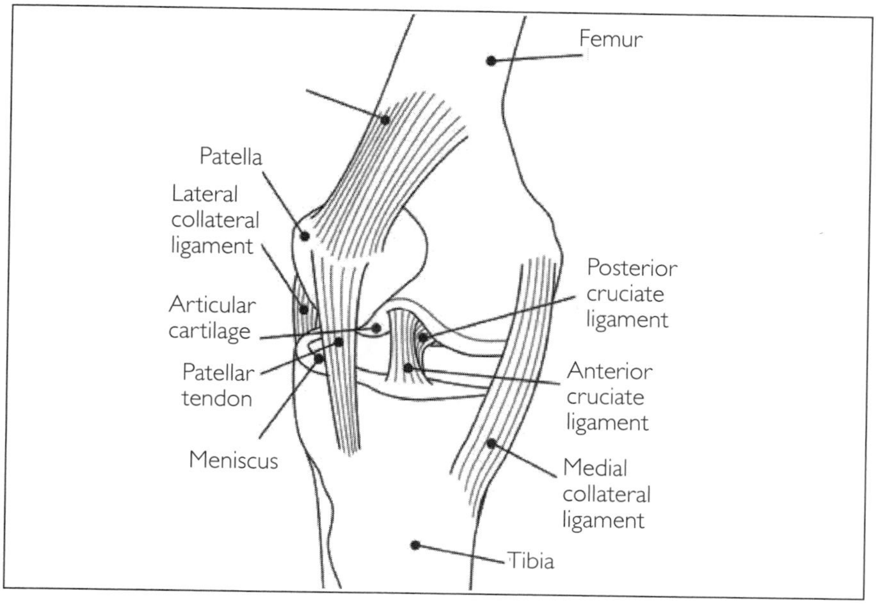

The knee is a weight-bearing joint with a complex structure. Millions of people visit orthopedic doctors every year due to knee problems. The ACL, one of four ligaments that supports the knee, is commonly injured—especially in women. This type of damage can occur from improperly landing after a jump, running too hard or too long, or insufficiently warming up. Adapted from http://www.niams.nih.gov/hi/topics/sports_injuries/Sports Injuries.htm.

Overtraining

Some athletes who train in excess develop what is called the *overtraining syndrome*, or *staleness*,[11] and experience physical and psychological problems such as fatigue, amenorrhea (in women), sleep disturbance, weight loss, and depression, as well as a decrease in performance. Unfortunately, many believe that a decline in performance due to staleness is a result of not training hard enough and will increase their workouts, which in reality, makes the problem *worse*. The solution is to reduce both the intensity of training and take some time off, as well as receive medical and psychological treatment.

We should note that child and adolescent athletes can also suffer from the overtraining syndrome. A multicultural study investigated this problem in adolescent swimmers and nearly 35% reported symptoms characteristic of staleness.[12] Given the potential health risks associated with the overtraining syndrome, coaches of youth sports and parents should be conscious of these symptoms in order to identify a problem early on, and intervene by helping the young athlete appropriately decrease training.

Athletes who are tempted to overtrain often rationalize that they *must* in order to excel. A recent study of Norwegian elite athletes representing 66 events and sports would suggest otherwise. These individuals averaged a reasonable 13.2 hours of training per week.[13] More evidence for balanced training levels comes from the previous example of Roger Bannister, who was the first person to run a mile in under four minutes. At the time, he was in medical training and therefore only able to train for less than an hour a day, five or six days a week. Furthermore, he did *not* train during the five days prior to his record-setting run. Bannister's example is proof positive that more training is not necessarily better.

> The overtraining syndrome, or staleness, leads to fatigue, depression, and decreased athletic performance. The solution is rest and recovery.

Mood Disturbance

The idea that exercise can improve one's mood is generally accepted. Ironically, the opposite appears to be true for some athletes, with elevations in mood disturbance corresponding to peaks in training.[14] That is to say, for these individuals an increase in training can *cause* mood swings, including depression, anxiety, or irritability, whereas a reduction can improve their mental state. Using the Profile of Mood States,[15] which measures specific factors (tension, depression, anger, vigor, fatigue, and confusion), the most frequent and greatest change for stale athletes is in depression scores. Athletes, coaches, and other sport personnel need to recognize that mood changes corresponding with increased training not only negatively impact performance, but might also be an early sign that an athlete is at risk for the overtraining syndrome. In the previously mentioned multicultural study of adolescent swimmers, stale swimmers reported more mood swings than the healthy group, which supports this idea.

Ultra-Endurance Athletes

In recent years we have seen the advent of ultra sports challenges, such as the Ironman competition. Ultra competitions are held in walking, swimming, and cycling, but in no area has this movement been more pronounced than in "ultramarathons"— running events that are longer than the traditional 26.2 miles. In North America alone there are more than 30 races that cover at least 100 miles. Many involve harsh environmental conditions to make the challenge even more difficult. A prime example is the Badwater Ultramarathon, a 135-mile race through Death Valley, California, that finishes halfway up Mount Whitney and usually takes place in July when the heat is most severe.

These types of races appear to be attracting more and more runners, many of whom are in their 30s, 40s, and 50s. The Western States Endurance Run in California started in 1977 with 14 runners (only three finished); but, the 2006 Run drew 399 runners (210 finished). And there would be even more participants if the Run did not require that competitors complete qualifying races.

Based on many of the criteria that we discussed in Chapter Three, ultra-endurance athletes are engaging in unbalanced, if not unhealthy, exercise. We mention them here because they are not simply individuals who are exercising too much. One also has to wonder about their daily lives. The time required to train adequately for and participate in such a competition would make having a normal life with a job and satisfying relationships difficult, as these individuals might do a 50-mile run on a typical training day, which could require 8 hours or more to complete. That much training would not leave much time for work, sleep, family, and a social life. Additionally, the medical risks for this group are apt to be considerable, especially when it comes to older ultra athletes and bone loss (58% of the finishers in the 2006 Western States Run were at least 40 years old and 18% were at least 50).

Despite the risk of compromised health, ultra-endurance athletes have an appetite for more—more mileage, more hours, more severe conditions. Where does it end? Is it enough only when the majority of the competitors cannot finish a race, or serious injuries or even deaths occur? The theme of this book is *balance*, and it is difficult to see any sort of balance in ultra-endurance sports. If anything, they are *intentionally* out of balance to the extreme, embracing the dubious maxim, "That which does not kill me, makes me stronger."[16]

Special Treatment Considerations for Competitive Athletes

Sometimes it is difficult to identify unhealthy or unbalanced exercise in athletes, but Table 4.2 offers several warning signs. Any one sign or symptom is not, in and of itself, indicative of a problem. However, regardless of age or level of training, if you see yourself on this checklist, you may need professional help. This might involve the support of a *treatment team,* which might include a medical doctor, counselor or therapist, dietitian/nutritionist, coach or trainer.

TABLE 4.2. Signs and Symptoms of Unhealthy or Unbalanced Exercise in Competitive Athletes

- Exercise is the individual's primary means of coping

- Exercise occurs despite injury

- Withdrawal effects (i.e., sleep and appetite disturbance, negative shift in mood, decreased concentration, etc.) occur when exercise is withheld

- Overuse injuries

- Stress fractures

- Menstrual irregularity in women or a decrease in testosterone levels in men

- Loss of bone density

- Decreased immunity

- Frequent colds and/or upper respiratory tract infections

- Inflexibility of exercise schedule (i.e., will not alter schedule; will not decrease exercise; will not NOT exercise)

- Decrease in sport performance

- "Overtraining Syndrome" (Staleness)

Unhealthy exercise is often part of an eating disorder, which is all too common in some sports. For this reason, unhealthy exercise by an athlete with an eating disorder will be used to illustrate issues related to the modification (treatment) of such exercise. The treatment team should strive to express empathy and compassion for an athlete's situation. Athletes have special issues, pressures, and concerns, and everyone needs to understand and appreciate this unique perspective. The sport may be an integral part of their identity and, in some cases, the primary or only source of self-esteem. Healthcare professionals need to realize this fact in order to best assist the athlete in finding a balance.

Too often athletes with eating and exercise problems are told that they must give up their sport temporarily or sometimes permanently. As a consequence, many leave treatment prematurely to continue with their workouts and do not return until their difficulties have worsened to the point that they have no alternative but to reluctantly seek help again. The question of whether an athlete seeking balance should continue to train and compete while in treatment will inevitably arise. The safe answer would be to stop all activity until recovered, and in many cases this is the best course to take. For example, symptoms suggesting vulnerability to sudden death should be taken very seriously and therefore sport participation must be discontinued.

However, other cases are not so clear cut. For example, say you are in treatment for an eating disorder, but have been evaluated medically and psychologically and found not to be at increased risk by participating in your sport. Should you be allowed to train and compete? Although the issues can be quite complex, there are actually several qualified reasons why the answer might still be yes. First, as we mentioned previously, being an athlete may be your primary identity and/or only source of self-esteem. If so, taking you out of this environment could actually create more problems than it solves. You might become depressed, lose more weight, or engage in other dangerous behaviors more often. Second, allowing you to remain with a team might provide the opportunity to be close to other players and give a needed sense of attachment and support. Third, if you are not allowed to train and compete, you might go against medical advice and exercise in secret. By allowing continuation, your exercise can be more readily monitored and, if necessary, controlled by appropriate sport personnel (coaches, athletic trainers, etc.). Fourth, allowing physical activity may make it easier to make the necessary or appropriate eating and weight changes. Fifth, competition can be used as motivation to make progress in treatment.

A final stipulation involves the safeguards that need to be in place. The benefit of continued training must outweigh medical and psychological risks. In other words, you must be in treatment, progressing, and complying with a list of health maintenance criteria, such as eating enough calories to maintain a proper energy balance given the training. (For more detailed information, see Sherman and Thompson.[17, 18])

Weight Loss and Athletic Performance

Earlier we alluded to a common belief in the sport world that a reduction in body weight or body fat will improve athletic performance. Many individuals will attempt to become leaner through unsupervised dieting and/or increased training, and these activities are often overlooked as being problematic. However, dieting is the primary precursor to an eating disorder and although not all who diet will develop one, many will. Athletes should *never* chance developing an eating disorder for the *possibility* of improving their skills. Nothing is more important than physical and emotional well-being, and good health and nutrition are requirements for superior athletic performance. Additional information about issues related to weight loss and athletics can be found in the *NCAA Coaches Handbook: Managing the Female Athlete Triad.*[19]

> Weight loss does not necessarily improve athletic performance.

This subject of weight loss is controversial. Although some research supports the idea that reduced body weight or body fat will enhance sport performance, it is certainly not definitive. While a few athletes do see improvements, for many the effect is negligible or, in fact, *negative*. We have worked with athletes who lost too much weight, lost it too rapidly, or lost it through unhealthy means, such as unbalanced training. They were physically weak and fatigued and sometimes malnourished and dehydrated. Weight loss in wrestlers has resulted in decreases in strength, anaerobic power, anaerobic capacity, and aerobic power. [20] We have also treated athletes who were so psychologically upset by the weight loss process that any potential positive effect was more than offset by the emotional turmoil they experienced. Clearly, having eating disordered thoughts makes it more difficult to reach one's potential or handle pressure, both of which are essential for success in sports. Fortunately, once we return patients to a more normal eating and exercise regimen, weight and strength are regained and performance typically improves.

There are many ways to improve without resorting to the risky business of dieting or overtraining, such as using visualization and mental preparation to sharpen focus, relaxation training to manage anxiety, and a host of other mental skills (i.e., positive self-talk, goal setting, etc.) that can be used to improve or increase motivation, concentration, confidence, and preparation for competition.

Notes

1. *significantly in recent years.* Raglin, J. D., & Wilson, G. S. (2000). *Overtraining in athletes;* In Y. L. Hanin (Ed.), *Emotions in Sport* (pp. 191-207). Champaign, IL: Human Kinetics.

2. *individuals with anorexia nervosa.* Thompson, R. A., & Sherman, R. T. (1999). "Good athlete" traits and characteristics of anorexia nervosa. Are they similar? *Eating Disorders: The Journal of Treatment and Prevention, 7,* 181-190.

3. *"the female athlete triad."* American College of Sports Medicine, (1997). Position stand: The female athlete triad. *Medicine and Science in Sports and Exercise, 29,* i-ix.

4. *low energy availability.* Loucks, A. B. Energy availability, not body fatness, regulates reproductive function in women. *Exercise and Sport Sciences Reviews, 31,* 144-148.

5. *15.2% of the nonathletes.* Torstveit, M. K., & Sundgot-Borgen, J. (2005), The female athlete triad exists in both elite athletes and controls. *Medicine & Science in Sports & Exercise, 37,* 1449-1459.

6. *from low energy availability.* Loucks, A. B. Energy availability, not body fatness, regulates reproductive function in women. *Exercise and Sport Sciences Reviews, 31,* 144-148.

7. *International Olympic Committee Medical Commission's Position Stand.* International Olympic Committee Medical Commission (2005), Position stand on the female athlete triad. Available: www.multimedia.olymic.org/pdf/en_report_917.pdf.

8. *volume threshold of training:* De Souza, M. J., & Miller, B. E. (1997). The effect of endurance training in reproductive function in male runners. *Sports Medicine, 23,* 357-374.

9. *National Osteoporosis Foundation (NOF):* Osteoporosis: Men. Available: www.nof.org/men.

10. *bone loss is greater.* Andersen, A. E., Wilson, T., & Schlechte, J. (2000). Osteoporosis and osteopenia in men with eating disorders. *The Lancet, 355,* 1967-1968.

11. *overtraining syndrome, or "staleness."* Raglin, J. D., & Wilson, G. S. (2000). *Overtraining in athletes.* In Y. L. Hanin (Ed.). *Emotions in Sport* (pp. 191-207). Champaign, IL: Human Kinetics.

12. *characteristic of staleness.* Raglin, J., Sawamura, S., Alexiou, S., Hassmen, P., & Kentta, G. (2000). Training practices and staleness in 13–18-year-old swimmers: A cross-cultural study. *Pediatric Exercise Science, 12,* 61-70.

13. *hours training per week.* Torstveit, M. K., & Sundgot-Borgen, J. (2005). The female athlete triad: Are elite athletes at increased risk? *Medicine & Science in Sports & Exercise, 37,* 184-193.

14. *peaks in training.* Raglin, J. D., & Wilson, G. S. (2000). *Overtraining in athletes.* In Y. L. Hanin (Ed.). *Emotions in Sport* (pp. 191-207). Champaign, IL: Human Kinetics.

15. *profile of mood states.* McNair, D. M., Lorr, M., & Dropplemann, L. F. (1992). Profile of mood states manual. San Diego, CA: Educational and Industrial Testing Services.

16. *makes me stronger.* Nietzsche, F. (1899). *The Twilight of the Idols.* (Translation by Duncan Large.) New York, NY: Oxford University Press Inc., New York.

17. *see Sherman and Thompson.* Sherman, R. T., & Thompson, R. A. (2001). Athletes with disordered eating: Four major issues for the professional psychologist. *Professional Psychology: Research and Practice, 32,* 27-33.

18. *see Sherman and Thompson.* Sherman, R. T., & Thompson, R. A. (2006). Practical use of the International Olympic Committee Medical Commission position stand on the female athlete triad: A case example. *International Journal of Eating Disorders, 39,* 193-201.

19. *Managing the Female Athlete Triad.* National Collegiate Athletic Association. (2005). *NCAA Coaches Handbook: Managing the Female Athlete Triad.* Indianapolis: The National Collegiate Athletic Association.

20. *and aerobic power.* Webster, S., Rutt, R, & Weltman, A. (1990). Physiological effects of a weight loss regimen practiced by college wrestlers. *Medicine and Science in Sports and Exercise, 22,* 229-234.

CHAPTER 5

Moderating Excessive Exercise

In this chapter, we first discuss guidelines and goals for moderating unhealthy or unbalanced exercise. We provide practical suggestions and recommendations for people who overdo it, with specific tips for compulsive and obligatory exercisers who need to decrease their activity. Finally, we explain the possible need for specialized assistance and how to find the appropriate healthcare professional.

Guidelines for Change

As previously noted, the primary guidelines for assessing whether or not one is exercising too much is if (1) physical or psychological health is compromised, or (2) the exercise regimen interferes with important activities such as school, work, or relationships. Once you've determined that you need to alter behaviors, there are several guiding principles. The basics for change include *awareness, positive thoughts and beliefs, motivation,* and *commitment.*

Awareness

Awareness is always the first step; you need to recognize *what* you are doing before you can change it. Most behaviors—healthy and unhealthy—serve one or more functions or purposes. Whether you realize it or not, they do something *for* you, such as help avoid, excuse, explain, or protect. For example, you may overexercise thinking that you are doing something beneficial without admitting that you are discontent in other areas of life. Exercise helps you to get away from problems or feelings. You may initially begin to do something for one obvious reason—such as, exercising to stay in shape. However, as you repeat an activity, it takes on more and more associations. The original purpose may even get blurred, and your behavior might eventually serve in so many ways that you may question whether to change it at all!

> A person must first be aware of the behavior that needs to be changed.

For example, Jay was a patient in his thirties, who on the advice of his primary care physician (PCP), started jogging for health reasons and to lose weight. After a month or two, he felt better, had more stamina, and received compliments from friends about how much "better" he looked. After his father had coronary bypass surgery, Jay increased his running with the idea that it might protect him from a similar fate. However, there were some unforeseen negative developments. Over the next couple of years, he was rejected in a romantic relationship (which he blamed on his appearance), got laid-off, and took a lower-paying job. His usual response was to run further. It allowed him to get outdoors and away from his troubles, plus he rationalized that he would avoid heart problems like his Dad. When he boasted to his PCP that he had daily two-hour workouts and ran for four to five hours on Saturdays or Sundays, the doctor wisely referred him for psychological counseling, where Jay worked on moderating his exercise and addressing his other issues in healthier ways.

Regardless of why someone becomes aware that his behavior is problematic, it is recognition that leads to change. Usually, awareness comes as a consequence of poor health or injuries, psychological problems, trouble in relationships, and difficulties at work or school.

Positive Thoughts and Beliefs

Another requirement for change is the belief that changing your behavior will be more beneficial than not changing it. You might think it's not worth the effort and say, "Oh, what difference will it make anyway?" However, rather than simply accepting this rhetorical question, answer it. Tell yourself what difference the change will make. Be specific. Make a list of what effects it could have on health, relationships, and life. Next, believe that change is possible. Make sure you are not using the false belief that you cannot change ("I can't do it, so why even try?") as a reason or excuse. This type of counterproductive thought must be avoided. You have to think it before you believe it. Practice thinking that you can change until you believe it.

Many people who undergo personal transformations, such as individuals in recovery programs, repeat *positive affirmations* to influence thinking. A common practice is to select a short phrase, write it down (over and over), and repeat it often throughout the day. Use the same affirmation or vary them from day to day. For example, to speak back to the internal voice that tells you to exercise more and more, when you need to do less, use words like these:

- "I am finally allowing my injuries to heal."

- "It feels good to rest."

- "By spending more time with my children than exercising, I'm being a better parent and am really getting to know them better."

- "By focusing more on my situation at work and less on the number of miles I'm running, I'm doing a much better job."

- "I'm improving my health by working out less."

Motivation

Motivation to change is vital. Whatever that motivation is, it must be stronger than the desire to stay the same. For example, one anorexic woman who hadn't menstruated since high school wanted to get pregnant, so she had to decrease her exercise and gain weight. In her case, the restrictive eating and overtraining masked a myriad of deep personal emotions. It was difficult for her to confront them rather than falling back on her usual, self-destructive ways of coping. However, she valued her marriage and goal to start a family above her desire to hide from the inner pain any longer.

Beginning in the 1980s and continuing into the new millennium, psychologists have been interested in how to evaluate a person's readiness to change. Prochaska and DiClemente have theorized that there are several stages to this process[1], called pre-contemplation, contemplation, preparation, action, and maintenance. Reading this book indicates being in the contemplation stage and somewhat motivated.

Commitment

Finally, you must stay committed. Lasting, positive change requires hard work, and it is easier to revert to old negative behaviors than to maintain a dedicated effort. For excessive exercisers, it may be more difficult not to workout than to run to the point of exhaustion. However, they obviously value hard work, and paradoxically must learn to apply their energy to decreasing or moderating their exercise.

> The objective is not to change quickly, but to change permanently.

Some people quit the change process because it isn't fast enough for them. You may need to adjust goals *and* thinking. The objective is not to change quickly, but to change permanently. Try to be patient. This may be difficult, especially for excessive exercisers, who as a group are generally not the most patient individuals. In fact, their need for stimulation or activity may play a role in how much they exercise. Some report that it is almost impossible to sit still. If this sounds familiar, you may need specialized assistance. At the end of this chapter we discuss when to consider, and how to find, professional help.

Beginning to Change

Change requires appropriate goals. We like the well-known, proven treatment objectives first proposed many years ago by Dr. Alayne Yates, a pioneer in the field of unhealthy exercise.[2] Yates proposed that the "end result of successful therapy is greater comfort with self, diminished activity coupled with greater enjoyment of the activity, and the ability to receive from others." If we substitute the word "change" for "therapy" we can paraphrase this as the desire to feel more psychologically comfortable, while decreasing the frequency, duration, and/or intensity of activity (exercise) and enjoying it more, and being able to relate well to others. We couldn't agree more. It emphasizes comfort, pleasure, and kinship. Who would disagree with that?

Now, let's look at where to begin the process of change. Obviously, exercise involves behavior. However, as we have already discussed, it also involves how you think, believe, perceive, and feel. So you must make adjustments in these areas as well.

It is important to evaluate attitudes and beliefs about exercise. You can do this in part by gathering and accepting accurate information on what is healthy and unhealthy in order to confront detrimental beliefs. For example, you might need to be completely honest regarding whether a regimen negatively affects health and/or everyday life. Although it sounds simple, assistance with this challenging task may need to come from an objective outsider, such as a loved one, honest friend, or therapist.

You must also increase body awareness while decreasing body obsessiveness. The body communicates through signs or symptoms, such as pain or fatigue. You need to recognize when you are helping your body and when you are hurting it. With failure to respond appropriately, your body will speak louder to get your attention. For example, runners who repeatedly abuse their knees or hips, ignoring pain and injury, will eventually have to face the orthopedic surgeon's scalpel. With failure to respond to an initial symptom, the condition is apt to worsen until you are willing or forced to deal with it.

As we stated before, excessive exercise meets one or more needs, so it is also important to learn to satisfy those needs in other ways. Otherwise, nothing is likely to change. One of the best ways to determine exactly what need is being met is by "withholding" the behavior and see what arises. Unfortunately, doing this can cause feelings of anxiety, depression, or guilt. What's more, individuals who are obligatory exercisers often cannot refrain from exercise long enough to determine the need that drives it. They become too impatient with the process, uncomfortable about changing routines, and give in to their compulsion. In this case, an evaluation by a psychotherapist experienced in dealing with such problems is warranted.

You must also address any unhealthy relationship between eating and exercise, such as increasing activity levels to compensate for, or legitimize, eating (or not eating, as in the case of anorexics). Simply put, the amount eaten should *not* be based on the level of exercise. If you continually feel the need to increase exercise to compensate for or "undo" the effects of eating "too many" calories, you should consult with an eating disorder specialist.

Strategies for Change

Before focusing specifically on changing an exercise behavior, some preparation and planning will increase the chances of success. The following recommendations can help collect and organize the information needed to target the behavior you want to change and make it easier to formulate specific plans to accomplish these goals. Even coming up with reasonable goals requires some forethought and investigation.

1. *Record* data on the behavior you want to change in an exercise log. Enter the type, frequency, duration, or amount of exercise done per day for a week. This establishes a baseline and allows you to be aware of what you are doing. Remember, keep it honest! The log should also include a column for comments, where you can jot down feelings and thoughts about the workouts. The format might look like the one in Table 5.1, which shows data recorded by a man who realized he was exercising too much and that it was influencing his life in a negative way. His willingness to provide accurate information allowed him to work with his therapist to devise strategies to successfully change his behavior.

TABLE 5.1. Personal Exercise Log: Baseline

Date	Type of exercise	Total time	Comments
Jan. 5	Running	2 hours	Less anxious but tired
Jan. 6	Running	2 hours	Feel proud
Jan. 7	Running Swimming	2 hr. 20 min 5 laps	Happy: lost one pound, but wife irritated with me for being late for party
Jan. 8	Running Swimming	2 hrs. 40 min. 10 laps	Calm but boss complained—task not done

Continued on next page

Jan. 9	Running	2 hrs. 50 min.	Left knee hurts, I want to increase
	Swimming	15 minutes	my laps
Jan. 10	Running	3 hour	Made goal! Brother mad because I
	Swimming	15 laps	didn't call him back
Jan. 11	Running	3 hrs. 10 min.	Knee hurts really bad, tired

Explanation: This is a baseline exercise log for Tom, a 40-year-old husband and father who began seeing a therapist because several of his life problems appeared to stem from his exercise. For example, Tom's family complained he was never available, his employer criticized him because his work was not completed on time, and his primary care physician had referred him to an orthopedist for his knee pain. The therapist asked Tom to keep a baseline exercise log for a week. By keeping a daily log and reviewing the immediate results, Tom could see how his exercise regimen was interfering with his work and family life and how it was affecting his health. He also realized that his exercise has positive effects, including a reduction in anxiety and a sense of accomplishment. He agreed to work toward a more moderate exercise regimen in order to achieve an exercise balance.

2.   *Research and apply* information about the behavior you want to change. Information that is accurate, reliable, and scientifically-based will help lead to success.

In a position stand[3], the American College of Sports Medicine (ACSM) makes the following recommendations for "the quantity and quality of training for developing and maintaining cardiorespiratory fitness, body composition, muscular strength and endurance, and flexibility in the healthy adult."

For cardiorespiratory fitness and body composition, the ACSM recommends 3–5 days per week with a training intensity of 55–90% maximum heart rate. (Ninety percent of maximum heart rate would be for very healthy, well-conditioned competitive athletes. For anyone else, however, we don't recommend exceeding 80% of maximum heart rate.) The duration should be 20–60 minutes of continuous or intermittent aerobic activity; in other words, the exercise can be performed in one session or a number of periods of at least 10 minutes per session throughout the day. These types of activities include walking/hiking, running/jogging, cycling, cross-country skiing, aerobic dance, rowing, swimming, skating, stair climbing, or sports, such as tennis, basketball, soccer, or volleyball.

The ACSM states that, "resistance training should be an integral part of an adult fitness program," and recommends 2–3 days per week of doing multiple sets of strengthening exercises, such as weight training.

ACSM also says that flexibility training should be incorporated into fitness programs and stretching should be performed a minimum of 2–3 days per week.

The American Council on Exercise (ACE) offers additional guidelines[4] for avoiding overuse injuries especially from running, but applicable to other types of exercise as well. ACE suggests to "always follow a relatively 'hard' day of exercising with an easier day" and incorporating an occasional "easy" week into your regimen, "Contrary to what some people believe, more is not always better...exercising too much substantially increases your chances of sustaining an overuse injury. Remember: Exercise quality is usually more important than quantity."

> A complete fitness program includes aerobics, resistance training, and stretching.

If you are not in training for athletic competition and the workouts exceed the recommendations of ACSM and ACE—or just plain, good sense—consider changing your routine. Glenn Gaesser, a noted exercise physiologist, proposes that people should exercise[5] an average of 20 minutes per day for good health, especially those who are just starting an exercise program. For more excellent information on this topic, visit the following websites: American College of Sports Medicine (www.acsm.org) and American Council on Exercise (www.acefitness. org/getfit/).

3. *Identify* the aspects of the exercise behavior to change. Examples might include changing the type of exercise (running to cross training), decreasing the frequency (7 times per week to 5), the duration (90 minutes to 60), and/or the intensity (85% of maximum heart rate to 70%).

With regard to maximum heart rate, let's say that you want to decrease the intensity of your exercise. Say you determine that 70% of your maximum heart rate would be a healthy target range. You would then subtract your age from 220 (this is a constant that is used for computation) and compute 70% of that number to determine 70% of your maximum heart rate. For example, if you are 40 years old, the calculation would be (220 - 40) x 0.70 = 126 beats per minute. Thus, you would aim to maintain your heart rate at 126 beats per minute or less while exercising to successfully decrease the intensity of the workout.

If you exercise for excessive periods of time, try to be honest about it. Most health and sports medicine groups recommend no more than 60 minutes at a time. If you exceed that recommendation, then you are probably exercising for reasons other than health. Unless you are a competitive athlete, you are most likely not working to improve a sport-related skill. Ask yourself: If I am not exercising for my health or competition, then why am I exercising so much? If you can determine the reasons for overexercising, then you will have a better sense about motivation and needs. This might help you meet your needs in a different way to decrease your dependence on exercise.

4. *Set reasonable goals.* Aim for gradual rather than abrupt change. Slow and steady progress both feels less intense and gives you and your body more time to adjust physi-

cally and psychologically to a new regimen. Write down goals, breaking them down to short-term and long-term. For example, a long-term goal would be decreasing the duration of daily exercise from two hours to one. Your short-term goal would be to reduce exercise sessions by 15 minutes per week. At first, decrease exercising from 2 hours to 1 hour 45 minutes and stay at that level for the first week. If you're successful, reduce your routine another 15 minutes for the next week, continuing this gradual process until the goal of one hour is reached. By systematically reducing the duration of exercise in small amounts, you will have gradually modified behavior, hopefully with a minimum of difficulty and discomfort. Practicing this new level of exercise duration should begin to feel more comfortable both psychologically and physically.

However, if you are unsuccessful at first, try cutting off 5 minutes every 2–3 days. If reducing even small amounts is not possible, more drastic measures are necessary. In fact, there may be a need to stop exercising completely and eventually resume at short durations. If you can neither decrease nor stop exercising, professional help is needed.

5. *Talk with someone* you trust about the changes you want to make and the strategies you want to try. When intentions are verbalized, it gives them life and strengthens resolve. Actually, you would probably benefit from outside input in determining goals and might seek assistance from an athletic trainer, therapist, or good friend. If there are health issues, start by talking with a primary care physician. Keep this person informed of goals and progress. This approach adds an element of accountability. If you pick someone who will be firm, honest, and supportive, then this person can help protect you from yourself. That is, your reasons, excuses, or rationalizations for not progressing with your change can be challenged. Additionally, instruct this person to offer praise when you do well, because positive reinforcement is a great motivator and can help you stay on track.

One way to reduce exercising for excessive periods of time is to have a partner, someone who will not only help you stay within a reasonable time limit, but also make the activity a social experience. If you'd rather not have a partner, ask yourself why. Could it have anything to do with your need to be in control? You might think that including another person will interfere with your workout or slow you down, but maybe this is exactly the reason why you *need* an exercise partner—to change your behavior and routine.

6. *Recognize* how you feel emotionally and physically. Try to be positive about your feelings. For example, if changing makes you anxious, take comfort that anxiety is part of the process and will eventually subside. Congratulate yourself for taking better care of your body. Praise yourself for having the fortitude to attempt altering unhealthy behavior despite the anxiety, because it indicates commitment to change as well as toughness and resolve. Remind yourself that there have been other situations when anxiety or fear were encountered, yet you persevered in spite of those feelings.

Such situations not only require commitment and toughness, they also require courage. Remember that courage is not the absence of fear, but rather doing what you need to do *despite* the fear. Even if you initially have some emotional turmoil as a result of decreasing your exercise, focus on how much better your body feels. Always be aware of and acknowledge the positives. Does your body feel less tired? Stronger? Rested? Allowing yourself to be aware of bodily feelings and sensations is reinforcing and can help motivate you to continue your quest for change.

> Positive reinforcement is a great motivator and can help you stay on track.

One good way to be in touch with your feelings is to regularly write in a journal. Some people routinely spend every morning and evening recording their thoughts. You might write daily goals to start the day, and at night reflect on the events and feelings that occurred. Also use your journal during times of stress, for example, when you might otherwise be exercising.

7. *Relax!* One of the hardest things a high-energy person can do is to do nothing at all; and yet, slowing down is absolutely essential for individuals who must decrease their activity. For someone who is constantly moving, sitting still and becoming centered on her own quiet inner self is tremendously worthwhile. One way to do this is through meditation, which is a component of numerous recovery programs. One simple way to meditate is by sitting quietly for 10–30 minutes with eyes closed while focusing on the breath coming in and going out. When thoughts arise, let them drift by while returning attention to breathing. Eventually, with practice, the thoughts subside and you discover inner peace. This is just one way to meditate—there are many others, any of which is beneficial. Meditating for a period of time that might otherwise be spent exercising is an excellent substitution. In fact, it may be as challenging to increase meditation time as to decrease exercise, but the rewards will be significant.

While mediation is a formal relaxation activity, there are other effective ways to relax, such as watching the sunset, carefully listening to music, taking a hot bath, or engaging in a hobby.

8. *Support yourself.* Don't be hard on yourself if expectations are not met on your first attempt. Berating yourself is never helpful; try to stay positive. Remember, you didn't learn to walk in a day. But staying positive does not mean lying to yourself or denying the truth. Review your steps and acknowledge where you fell short, but "balance" it with positives. Focusing only on the negative is apt to lead to frustration and decreased motivation. Be objective and try to determine what necessary adjustments are needed for more success next time.

Many people can succeed if they stay committed and motivated, but others find that professional support helps them get past obstacles. As therapists, we assume that it is a sign of strength—not weakness—to ask for help.

Remember Tom? Here's his exercise log after six months of adapting healthier patterns of exercise:

TABLE 5.2. Personal Exercise Log: After 6 Months

Date	Type of exercise	Total time	Comments
July 1	Running Stretching	45 minutes 15 minutes	Worked up a good sweat Muscles felt good
July 2	Weights Swimming	30 minutes 30 minutes	Feel pumped and awake!
July 3	Running Stretching	30 minutes 5 minutes	Didn't have much time today. Felt a little frustrated.
July 4	Played softball	90 minutes	Not much of a workout, but had a lot of fun! First time in years I didn't enter a half-marathon.
July 5	Running Stretching	45 minutes 15 minutes	Glad to be back into my normal routine.
July 6	Weights Running Stretching	30 minutes 45 minutes 15 minutes	Kind of overdid it, because I'd felt deprived on the 4th. I need to watch it!
July 7	No exercise	Took a rest day.	

Explanation: Tom continued keeping an exercise log and noting his feelings. Instead of running so much anymore, he used cross training, including resistance and flexibility training. He remained tempted to exercise more like he used to, but he recognized the warning signs and took measures to ensure that he would not fall back into old, excessive routines.

Strategies for Specific Exercise Problems

In Chapter Three, we differentiated between compulsive and obligatory exercise and explained in what ways working out can be like an addiction. Although anyone who suffers from these tendencies should practice the strategies for change that we've discussed in this chapter, individuals with these specific problems usually need to do even more to change their behaviors.

If you are a compulsive exerciser—someone who has to do the same exercise for the same amount of time at the same time every day—vary the type of exercise. For example, if you are a runner, substitute weight training every other day. Eventually, progress to cross-training and rest days. You might try scheduling exercise, writing on a calendar which workouts to do. Put some rest days in, as well.

Compulsive behaviors are often used to manage fear and/or anxiety and usually involve issues related to control. Although alternating types of exercise may not seem to meet the same needs as the original exercise regimen, this will actually give you more control or "degrees of freedom." Again, keep in mind that compulsive behaviors are often difficult to change, and professional help may be needed.

Sometimes compulsive exercise is part of an obsessive compulsive disorder (OCD) and may require specific treatment. Cognitive-behavior therapy might include learning relaxation techniques, as well as restructuring one's thinking, to help patients tolerate the anxiety while they gradually decrease the compulsion—in this case, either the intensity or duration of exercise. If you do not relent and exercise, which can make the problem worse, the anxiety will eventually dissipate. An experienced therapist is needed, but improvement is usually effective and long lasting.

Another approach to OCD is the use of medications called selective serotonin reuptake inhibitors (SSRIs) such as fluoxetine or sertraline, or a tricyclic drug called clomipramine. Although often very helpful, the compulsive symptoms may recur if the medication is discontinued. Of course, these medications must only be used under the supervision of a physician, usually a psychiatrist.

If you are an obligatory exerciser, then you believe that skipping exercise is *not* an option. You definitely need outside support! Frankly, the world will not collapse if the exercise behavior is changed. You might have to face uncomfortable feelings and confront emotional pain that have been avoided, but a therapist would be able to help with that. Professional assistance is especially important if you continue to exercise while sick, injured, and/or are going against medical advice. At the very least, try enlisting the help of a friend or loved one, explaining your fears about changing or eliminating an exercise obsession. Ask him or her to spend time with you so that you won't work out. Regardless of whom you turn to for support, understand and accept that the behavior has gotten out of hand and needs to change.

Sometimes using the change strategies we have outlined or getting help from family or friends is not enough. You may need a detailed analysis to determine all the factors contributing to the problem and to locate ways of altering the unhealthy drive to exercise. There may be associated psychiatric problems such as bipolar disorder or various types of anxiety disorders influencing behavior. If you are unable to change obligatory exercise, then a psychiatric evaluation should be the next step.

More Considerations for When to Seek Professional Help

Many people are able to change behavior through self-help work, like journal writing, meditation, goal setting, and other suggestions we've discussed. However, sometimes the task of changing one's routine is simply too difficult, complicated, or overwhelming for an individual. This is especially the case when the behavior has been practiced for a long period of time and serves several functions or purposes. If you are unsuccessful at changing on your own, then it is time to get professional help. We encourage you to recognize the need for assistance as a positive move, a way of making life better.

Professional assistance can come from many different disciplines. Emotionally-based problems would be faced by working with a psychiatrist, psychologist, social worker, or other mental health specialist. Physical concerns would be directed to a primary care physician, who would refer specialists (cardiologist, orthopedic surgeon, etc.) depending on your needs. If you need help in designing an exercise program, talk to an athletic trainer, physical therapist, exercise physiologist, or coach. Dietary issues should be discussed with a doctor or a registered dietitian. In many instances, a treatment team made up of a combination of these professionals is the best approach.

> Recognize the need for assistance as a positive move, a way of making your life better.

Consult a therapist or other mental health professional when encountering one or more of the following circumstances while attempting to change:

1. *Excessive exercise is out of control.* In order for an individual to change a behavior, he or she must have at least some degree of control. Obvious warning signs would be continuing to exercise despite sustaining an injury, such as a stress fracture, or ignoring (or denying) signs or symptoms of possible serious medical complications, such as chest pain, during exercise. Others would be continuing to increase the intensity, frequency, and/or duration of exercise beyond what is necessary or recommended for age or health status. In such a situation, you may be telling yourself that you are not exercising often, long, or hard enough. Most likely, you are not listening to your body.

2. *Attempts to change cause emotions that are difficult to manage.* As mentioned previously, excessive exercise is apt to be related to, or used to, manage unpleasant or difficult emotions. Therefore, attempts to change may evoke emotions that are overwhelming. If, for example, excessive exercise is being used to manage or hide feelings of depression, changing the behavior may leave the person too depressed to cope effectively. If change produces a condition that is more difficult than the one created by excessive exercise, professional help is indicated.

3. *Attempts to change bring on other maladaptive behaviors or symptoms.* Attempting to change may bring on not only unpleasant emotions, but also unwanted changes in other behaviors, such as sleep patterns or eating habits. A marked increase or decrease in the amount one sleeps and/or eats is often attributable to feelings of depression or anxiety. Some people resort to alcohol or drugs to help them cope, in which case professional help is needed to understand the underlying issues. There are many proven treatments for these kinds of problems.

4. *Attempts to reduce exercise results in food deprivation.* Some excessive exercisers will eat less if they begin to exercise less. At first this might sound reasonable, but it can, in fact, be a serious problem. In reality, there are situations in which a person should eat less if he or she does not exercise as much as usual. But in this particular case, the individual eats less not because she needs fewer calories but because she feels that she has not "earned" or "does not deserve" the calories. She uses exercise to "undo" the effects of eating by creating a negative energy balance in order to lose or not gain weight. Not surprisingly, eating disorder patients often will not allow themselves to eat at all if they feel that they have not exercised enough (which is actually too much). Consultation with an eating disorder treatment specialist would be appropriate.

5. *Change negatively affects significant others.* Sometimes a change in one person can evoke changes in others. That is, family members or close friends may react to the effects of your behavioral change. For example, a husband and father may affect the household stress level by how he relates to his family. Excessive running takes him out of the house and away from the family for long periods of time. His routine allows him to reduce some of his tension, which in turn keeps the stress level lower for other family members. If he then significantly reduces his exercise, he will be home more and won't be as relaxed. In this way, his family may actually "need" his excessive exercise as much, or more, than he does. In a situation such as this, a referral to a good family therapist is probably warranted for the sake of improving family relationships and responsibilities.

6. *Attempts to decrease excessive exercise may actually increase it.* Sometimes attempting to change can produce a paradoxical or reactive effect. For some people, just thinking about changing their behavior causes them to feel a need to increase it. In their eyes, the prospect of changing, or taking away, the behavior may actually increase its value. Such situations might include a person who is planning to begin a diet tomorrow so he will eat more today, or a person who is going to quit smoking so he smokes more than usual before buckling down. Given this increase in the target behavior, a professional may need to set up your change process so as not to produce negative effects.

7. *Attempts to change are met with continued avoidance.* In this case, repeated attempts to change are never realized because you continue to find reasons not to start the process. Examples of avoidance are familiar: "I'm too busy." "I'll start next week." "I'm waiting until it feels right." "I'm waiting until I'm more motivated." "This is so important I want to wait until I can give it my full attention." These examples are excuses or rationalizations—the opposite of balanced thinking. If one really wants to change but can't seem to get started, a cognitive therapist or life coach can help you get beyond a particular set of avoidance strategies.

8. *Attempts to change are continuously met with self-sabotage.* Some people briefly work at change and then create a situation in which they are bound to fail. For example, they may set goals that are unrealistic or give up after having a relapse. As we have discussed previously, exercise behavior probably serves one or more purposes or functions, and as a result, you may have many unconscious reasons not to change. Psychologically, you may be motivated to maintain the status quo because it's comfortable and undermines any attempts to change. Awareness is the first step in changing a behavior. Thus, you may need a professional to assist in increasing, maintaining, or using awareness to avoid sabotaging efforts to change.

9. *Repeated attempts to change are unsuccessful.* Change is difficult, because it is usually easier to stay the way you are. If you really want to change, don't frustrate yourself with repeated unsuccessful change attempts. Admit that help is needed and contact someone who can assist in achieving your goals.

Perhaps you are the type of person who resists professional help because you want to "do it yourself." Understand that a therapist is not going to make the change for you anymore than a coach runs laps for you. Any change that occurs is still accomplished by *you*. "Doing it yourself" does not have to mean "doing it alone."

Notes

1. *several stages to this process.* Prochaska, J, DiClemente (1982). Transtheoretical therapy: toward a more integrative model of change. *Psychotherapy: Theory, Research and Practice* (pp. 276-288).

2. *pioneer in the field of unhealthy exercise:* Yates, A. (1991). *Compulsive Exercise and the Eating Disorders: Toward an Integrated Theory of Activity.* New York: Brunner/Mazel.

3. *In a position stand.* American College of Sports Medicine, (1998). Position stand: The recommended quantity and quality of exercise for developing and maintaining cardiorespiratory and muscular fitness, and flexibility in healthy adults. *Medicine and Science in Sports and Exercise* 30.

4. *offers additional guidelines.* American Council on Exercise (2007). ACE FitnessMatters. Available: http://www.acefitness.org/fitfacts/fitnessqa_display.aspx?itemid=368.

5. *day of exercise.* Gaesser, G. (2002) *Big Fat Lies: The Truth about Your Weight and Your Health.* Carlsbad, CA: Gürze Books.

CHAPTER 6

Characteristics and Hazards of Insufficient Exercise

Earlier, we discussed the topic of overexercise; in this chapter, we look at the other side of the exercise balance—*under*exercise. Most people do not meet recommended physical activity levels, and these individuals are susceptible to problems with obesity and chronic illness. Regardless of the reasons for not exercising, there are negative physical and emotional consequences to a sedentary lifestyle.

Fewer than 50% of Americans exercise regularly[1] and 66% are overweight or obese.[2] The connection between these two statistics is obvious. A lack of physical activity is unhealthy, but there are obvious benefits to regular exercise, including improvements to cardiovascular, metabolic, bone, and psychological health. So, given the simple fact that exercise is healthy, why don't more people do it?

There are a limitless number of rationalizations for people to avoid exercising. Our society no longer requires us to do physical labor or walk long distances. We sit at our computers all day. There's never enough time. Physical education has been eliminated from school curricula. We spend too many hours in front of the television. Illness makes it difficult. Ask anyone with an excuse, and they will probably also say, "But I'd like to exercise more," or "I know I should, and I'm going to get started soon." They may mean well and have great intentions, but their procrastination and ambivalence make it hard for them to begin and maintain an exercise routine. However, resistance can be overcome.

For example remember Bill from Chapter 1, who has borderline diabetes mellitus and is 30 pounds overweight? Although his physician recommended an increase in physical activity, Bill was reluctant to begin an exercise program. Previous attempts at sticking to a workout schedule failed when he didn't lose weight, so he was reluctant to try again. However, Bill didn't realize that it takes significantly less exercise to lower blood sugar levels—thereby reducing his vulnerability to complications of diabetes mellitus—than to lose weight. Once he understood that he could have health benefits from a mild workout, it seemed less daunting.

What Is Underexercise or Insufficient Exercise?

Insufficient exercise is defined as a physical activity level that is occurring less than the frequency, intensity, and duration necessary to attain or maintain good cardiovascular health, fitness, flexibility, and strength appropriate to age, gender, and health status. As we pointed out in the last chapter, experts recommend moderately intense exercise for a minimum of 30 minutes per day, five days per week, on average, and for healthy adults anything less than that would fall into the unhealthy category.

Inadequate physical activity contributes to the development of several diseases, such as heart disease, adult onset diabetes mellitus, obesity, and depression, just to name a few. These diseases and difficulties have often been called *hypokinetic*, or low activity, diseases. A classic example of the development of a hypokinetic disease is illustrated by the Pima Indians.

Genetics and Environment Interaction: The Pima Indians

What happened to the Pima Indians who live in the Sonoran desert in southwestern Arizona is a prime example of the role physical activity plays in weight maintenance.[3] Prior to the 1920s, the Pima Indians were physically active farmers who worked in teams, moving from farm to farm. As a group, they appeared to be naturally thin and had one of the lowest rates of diabetes mellitus in the nation. With the advent of labor saving devices, their physical activity experienced a sharp decline. Today, they have *high*er rates of obesity and diabetes mellitus than any other ethnic group in the United States.[4] By 1995, 50% of Pima Indians between the ages of 30-64 had Type 2 diabetes mellitus, and in 95% of those cases the individual also suffered from obesity. In comparing the photographs of Pima Indians before and after the 1920s, their physical transformation is quite evident.

FIGURE 6.1. Pima Indian Farmer Prior to 1920

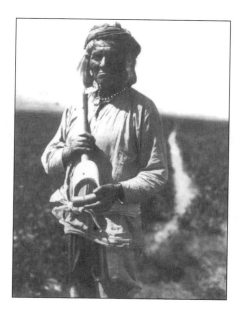

Before the 1920s, members of this ethnic group were generally thin and had very low rates of diabetes mellitus. From: *The Pima Indians: Pathfinders for Health, National Institute of Diabetes and Digestive and Kidney Diseases, NIH Publication No. 95-3821*. Used with permission.

Studies of the Pima Indians have contributed to the concept of a *thrifty genotype*.[5] Over several millennia, food supplies were scarce and obtaining food required large energy expenditures. Those individuals with genetic mutations resulting in fewer calories required to perform physical activities were more likely to survive. This mutation (or more likely a series of mutations) can take thousands of years to occur and resulted in what we call the thrifty genotype. However, after thousands of years of success, the advent of plentiful food and decreased physical activity quickly transformed this genetic advantage into a liability, especially for full-blooded Pima Indians, who have this gene. In the last two decades, sophisticated studies of this group have confirmed much of the thrifty genotype hypothesis. These studies show that a significant reason for the weight differences in this ethnic group is related to genetic factors regulating food intake and voluntary physical activity.[6] In other words, the Pima Indians from Arizona were genetically inclined to obesity when their manual labor diminished. This is further evident by looking at a remote group of Pima Indians from Mexico, who still live in the manner of their ancestors and have no problems with obesity or diabetes.

FIGURE 6.2. Present-day Pima Indian

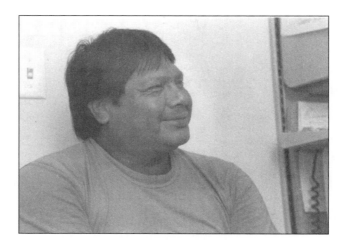

Because physical activity has declined precipitously since the 1920s and food is now abundantly available, about 75% of adult Pima Indians are now overweight or obese and 50% have diabetes mellitus. From: *The Pima Indians: Pathfinders for Health, National Institute of Diabetes and Digestive and Kidney Diseases, NIH Publication No. 95-3821.* Used with permission.

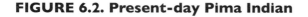

What Is Wrong with Insufficient Exercise or a Sedentary Lifestyle?

The answer to this question is found in a report by the Surgeon General (1996)[7] that looked at the role physical activity plays in preventing disease. The report concludes that the absence of regular exercise increases the risk of developing or dying from heart disease, non-insulin-dependent diabetes mellitus, hypertension, and colon cancer. It also concluded that underexercise is associated with less healthy bones, muscles, and joints, plus weight gain and symptoms of anxiety and depression.

Surprisingly, many people do not recognize the connection between the lack of adequate exercise and various diseases. One study[8] found that almost half of the U.S. college students surveyed did not realize that lack of exercise is associated with a greater risk for heart disease, hypertension, or diabetes mellitus. Interestingly, in many developed countries in Western Europe, more students recognized the connection between lack of exercise and physical complications. Not surprisingly, the rates of obesity in those countries are less than in the United States. However, in some of the developing nations in Eastern Europe, where fewer students recognize this connection than in the United States, the rate of physical illnesses associated with insufficient exercise and obesity is increasing rapidly.

Decreases in Physical Activity: A Global Problem

In developing countries, physical activity levels tend to decrease as more and more people move to the city, leaving fewer people to work at physically arduous rural jobs. For example, the Chinese population experienced dramatic changes in physical activity between 1989 and 1997.

FIGURE 6.3. Rapid Change in Physical Activity Levels in China

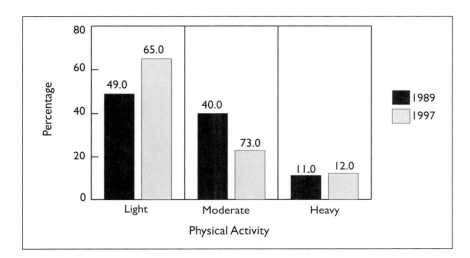

Declining physical activity is a global problem. This diagram shows how in China the level of physical activity of young adults declined dramatically in less than a decade. The increase in sedentary lifestyles is a contributing factor to the rise of obesity in countries throughout the world.

In 1989, 49% of urban Chinese adults aged 20–45 had light physical activity profiles. By 1997, the number had increased to 65%.[9] Once considered among the leanest populations, by 2002 "the obesity epidemic" hit China and more than 200 million people—over 17%—were overweight or obese. Although low by Western standards, this prevalence is steadily growing—most alarmingly among schoolchildren, whose rate increased 28 times between 1985 and 2000.[10] The rapid shift in activity levels, as well as changes in the types of foods consumed, are linked with greater levels of obesity.

Changes in physical activity and diet are occurring in developing countries throughout the world, and the consequences in terms of obesity and obesity-related illnesses may be even worse than in the United States or Western Europe for several reasons.[11] First, the changes often occur very rapidly, usually within a 10-year span. Second, because many people in developing counties were undernourished during fetal life, infancy, and childhood, the physiology of these individuals may have changed so that fewer calories are needed to maintain normal body functions. Then, when food becomes plentiful and less physical activity is required to survive, obesity may be a likely outcome.

Once a population recognizes the health risks associated with decreased physical activity and the increased consumption of high-calorie, high-fat foods, eating disorders appear or increase. For example, 25 years ago anorexia nervosa and bulimia nervosa were virtually unknown in China and other developing countries. Now, eating disorders in rapidly changing countries are not only prevalent, but on the rise.[12]

On the positive side, some Western European countries seem to have made strides in achieving a moderate balance. Physical activity (as opposed to scheduled exercise) in many of these countries is an integral part of life. For example, walking to the store or train station often occurs on a daily basis. Eating patterns also are different, with less focus on snacks or fast foods. The effect on obesity is significant. In France, for example, the rate of obesity is a mere 8.8%[13] compared to over 30% in the United States. However, even in Western Europe, challenges to this way of life are significant.[14]

Effect of Age, Gender, and Ethnicity

A 2004 report by the National Center for Health Statistics[15] states that there is a new trend of physical inactivity occurring in both younger and older Americans, and that the percent of individuals who do not exercise increases with age. According to this study, almost 40% of Americans over age 18 and more than 50% of adults 65 or older reported that they were not physically active during their leisure time. However, there is good news for even those who have not exercised for most of their lives: beginning an exercise program when you are older still can produce positive results in terms of improving health.

Gender also plays a role. In the report cited earlier, 40% of high school girls—as compared to 27% of high school boys—did not participate in the recommended amounts of exercise. In fact, women are less physically active in general than men of the same age.

Ethnicity, education, and socio-economic level are also related to physical health. Statistically, African-Americans and Hispanic-Americans engage in less leisure time activity than white Americans. Lower levels of physical activity are also associated with lower educational levels and lower socio-economic levels. Also, Americans with disabilities are less apt to be physically active.

Physical Consequences of Insufficient Exercise

Do people exercise less because of their medical conditions or are their diseases caused by lack of exercise? It's a chicken-and-egg proposition. Everyone's health is determined by genetics, age, environment, diet, and activity level. Although we cannot change our genetic proclivity for a certain level of physical activity, we can change how much we *choose* to exercise. By just adding a few minutes of exercise per day, people of all ages and sizes see improvements for most of the diseases that are related to a sedentary lifestyle. (In Chapter Nine we will provide more information related to exercise and chronic illness.)

The most common type of heart disease associated with insufficient exercise is *coronary heart disease.* This means that the arteries that supply the heart with oxygen (the coronary arteries) have become dangerously narrow from the deposit of plaque. The unfortunate result is often a myocardial infarction, which is commonly known as a heart attack. This is a serious event where part of the heart muscle that is supplied with oxygen by the coronary arteries actually dies.

Sometimes there is ischemia, or a diminished supply of oxygen to the heart, resulting in injury, but not death, of parts of the heart muscle. When this occurs the person may develop angina pectoris (periodic chest pain). Ultimately, the death or injury of heart muscle can result in severe functional impairments or death of the individual. However, exercise strengthens the heart muscle and increases its working capacity, lowers blood pressure, raises high density lipoprotein levels ("good" cholesterol), and lowers low density lipoprotein levels ("bad" cholesterol).

Another disease related to underexercise is *hypertension,* commonly known as high blood pressure. Contrary to popular belief, hypertension is a serious condition and should not be taken lightly. There are two parts to blood pressure measurement—the *systolic* and *diastolic* measures. The systolic pressure is the maximum pressure in an artery at the moment when the heart is beating and pumping blood through the body. The diastolic pressure is the lowest pressure in an artery in the moments between beats when the heart is resting. A health care professional inflates a blood pressure cuff on the upper arm while listening to an artery with a stethoscope. The cuff is then deflated and the systolic blood pressure is the first sound the doctor hears and the diastolic blood pressure is the second sound. The pressure detected is measured in millimeters of mercury, which is abbreviated as mmHg. This gives a common blood pressure reading such as 120/70 mmHg. Although it was once thought that an elevated diastolic blood pressure was the most dangerous, it is now known that an elevated systolic blood pressure is also dangerous.

The definition of "normal" blood pressure is changing and very small increases in blood pressure have recently been shown to be associated with dire consequences. Normal blood pressure is less than 120/80 mmHg.[16] Table 6.1 lists the major categories of blood pressure. When the blood pressure is in the pre-hypertensive range

(120-139/80-89mmHg) a doctor will probably recommend changes in lifestyle, usually including a recommendation to increase exercise.

TABLE 6.1. Blood Pressure Categories

- **Normal:** Less than 120/80 mmHg

- **Pre-hypertension:** 120-139/80-89 mmHg

- **Stage 1 Hypertension:** 140-159/90-99 mmHg

- **Stage 2 Hypertension:** 160 and above/100 and above mmHg

Another deadly disease that is associated with insufficient exercise is *diabetes mellitus,* a metabolic disorder in which the ability to oxidize (break down and use) carbohydrates (sugars and starches) is lost or compromised. As a result, blood levels of glucose, or blood sugar, increase. This elevated blood sugar is linked to many health complications, including coronary heart disease (which often leads to circulation problems in the legs and can lead to amputation), cerebral vascular accidents (strokes), blindness, and kidney failure. There are two major types of diabetes mellitus. *Type 1* usually begins in childhood or adolescence and is characterized by an absence of insulin production from the pancreas. Patients with Type 1 diabetes must have daily insulin injections. This type of diabetes mellitus is sometimes incorrectly called insulin-dependent diabetes, but patients with *either* Type 1 or Type 2 may require insulin. *Type 2* diabetes, which used to begin primarily in mid-life or later, is associated with insulin resistance; that is, the insulin that is available does not work as it should. Unfortunately, there has been a recent, dramatic increase of Type 2 diabetes in children, adolescents, and young adults,

> Modest increases in physical activity and small weight losses can significantly improve blood glucose levels in people with Type 2 diabetes mellitus.

which coincides with more childhood obesity and fewer physical education classes in our schools. However, it is encouraging that marked improvement in blood glucose levels often occurs after only a modest increase in physical activity and a relatively small weight loss. Therefore, diabetics who make small changes in their physical activity levels and food choices will usually see significant improvements in their health. Incidentally, in response to the rise in childhood obesity, some school districts are reinstating mandatory P.E. classes.

TABLE 6.2. Common Physical Consequences of Insufficient Exercise

- Coronary artery disease (e.g., heart attacks)

- Hypertension (high blood pressure)

- Cerebral vascular accidents (strokes)

- Increased risk of colon cancer

- Type 2 diabetes mellitus

- Osteoarthritis (joint deterioration)

- Osteopenia and Osteoporosis (loss of bone mass and/or density)

- Impaired muscle strength (which can lead to falls)

- Obesity

- Gallbladder disease

- Sleep apnea

- Certain types of cancer

Psychological Aspects of Insufficient Exercise: The Mind-Body Connection

The relationship between the mind and the body has been recognized since ancient times. Hippocrates, a Greek physician living around 400 B.C. and considered to be the Father of Medicine, observed, "Men ought to know that from the brain, and from the brain only, arise our pleasures, joys, laughter and jests, as well as our sorrows, pains, griefs, and fears. Through it, in particular, we think, see, hear…."[17] Aristotle, a philosopher and contemporary of Hippocrates, believed that the "Body and soul are reciprocally connected through the individual's temperament and consequently influence each other."[18] During the Middle Ages the mind-body question became a religious one and the separation of the body and mind became institutionalized. In the 1600s, French philosopher René Descartes formalized this division, or dichotomy, between mind and body as shown in his classic drawing of pain.[19]

FIGURE 6.4. Classic Representation of Pain by René Descartes

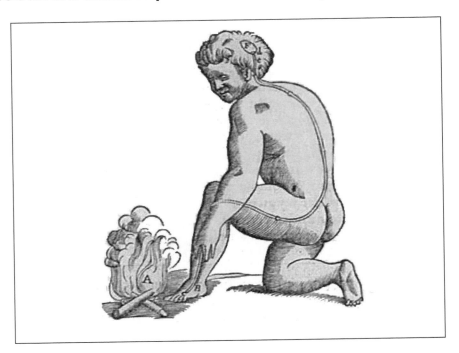

Descartes' drawing has come to symbolize the popular—yet inaccurate—belief that the mind and body are separate, which contributes to modern-day body image disturbances.

Due in large part to the long-standing influence of Descartes' work, which was reinforced by religious doctrine, the human body became conceptualized as mechanistic and reduced to elementary parts and systems for explanations of disease. It was not until the last 150 years this view was challenged. Perhaps the most influential challenge was by Sigmund Freud, who in 1923 concluded, "The ego is first and foremost a bodily ego."[20] By ego, Freud meant what is usually referred to as the mind, or the thinking, rational part of the brain. The implication of this principle is that the state of the body influences the thinking and feeling part of the brain and vice versa.

Achieving a moderate, healthy exercise regimen requires an integration of the *mind's* thinking and feeling parts and the *body's* activities. This integration of mind and body is crucial for anyone making life changes. In Chapter Three, we explained how overexercise affects mental and emotional health. Similarly, underexercise can be the result of an inability to cope with life's issues.

For example, Susan was a young woman in her late 20s who never worked out or participated in sports. An only child of two intellectual university professors, everyone thought of her as a "geek" and she got pushed into areas other than athletics. During adolescence, her father died after a long battle with cancer, and Susan became a sullen and depressed teenager. By the time we met her a few years ago, Susan had dropped out of graduate school, had never had a romantic relationship, and possessed generally low self-esteem. She couldn't sleep well and had become a binge eater, which brought her to our attention. We introduced exercise slowly while counseling her about her eating disorder. Through psychotherapy, her story emerged, and we addressed her emotional problems and the lack of balance between her intellect and activity. Susan did well in therapy, which helped her in many ways, and she also became an avid cyclist. The self-confidence she gained, combined with her improved strength, stamina, and enthusiasm for biking, transformed her into a powerful woman. Last summer, she recorded an amazing blog that chronicled a three-month, solo, cross-country bike trip.

Body Image and Insufficient Exercise

The way in which the mind and body are connected is evident by looking at the study of *body image*, which is the mental blueprint of one's body and is influenced by physical sensations—particularly touch and kinesthesia, the sensory experience of movement. Early childhood experiences with nurturing individuals (usually one's mother or father) significantly influence the way in which one's body is experienced. Adolescence is another important developmental period, and positive or negative events during this time can have enduring effects on self-perception. For example, adolescents who have been sexually abused may develop distorted feelings about themselves, and may learn to cope by fostering a conceptual division between mind and body. Some abused adolescents begin to overexercise in an effort to "punish" the body as a "re-enactment" of the sexual abuse they experienced. On the other hand, they may underexercise and gain weight as a way of "hiding" or "insulating" the body. These coping mechanisms illustrate some of the complexities in the mind-body relationship.

> Body image is the mental blueprint of one's body.

In recent years, there has been an explosion of interest in this topic and the emergence of new, and sometimes confusing or conflicting information. Part of the difficulty in interpreting these studies is that multiple methods have been used to evaluate different aspects of body image. Although the most popular tests of body image rely on sight, these tests may not capture the most important sensory aspects of body image, namely touch and kinesthesia. One commonly-used test is the Figure Rating Scale[21] shown in Figure 6.5.

FIGURE 6.5. Figure Rating Scale

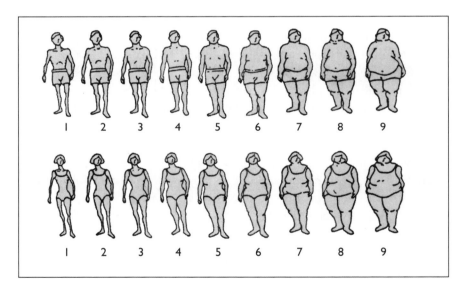

This scale is used to measure the way an individual perceives his or her body, or "perceptual aspect of body image." Used with permission from Stunkard et al, 1980.

In this test, the person is asked to choose the outline of the figure believed to be closest to his or her actual appearance, and then choose the figure that best approximates his or her desired appearance. The greater the difference between the actual and desired body shapes represents the extent of that person's body image disturbance. Although this test is helpful when it comes to measuring how someone *sees* his body, it does not assess the tactile or kinesthetic perceptual aspects of body image—the ways in which a person experiences bodily movements through space and time (such as walking). This part of body image is probably the most important determinant of body satisfaction even though it is the most difficult to measure. Body satisfaction is the attitudinal aspect of body image and has been measured in several tests. An example is the Body Parts Satisfaction Scale.[22] This scale consists of 24 items on body parts as well as overall appearance. Each item is rated on a 6-point Likert scale from "extremely dissatisfied" to "extremely satisfied."

The problem with these assessments is that they only measure either the perceptual aspects of body image (for example the visual assessment of one's body as in the Figure Rating Scale) or the attitudinal aspects of body image (as in the Body Parts Satisfaction Questionnaire). The division between mind and body is mirrored in these two tests. Several other tests have been developed that attempt to integrate measures of both the perceptual and attitudinal aspects of body image, but even the names of these tests reflect the absence of adequate words to describe the whole experience. Many use hyphenated phrases or cumbersome descriptions to try to convey the integration of mind and body, such as the "Multidimensional Body Self-Relations Questionnaire,"[23] the "Social Physique Anxiety Scale,"[24] and the "Physical Self-Efficacy Scale."[25]

The differences in these assessments reflect the complexity of body image, and some researchers have argued[26] that trying to create scales to measure beliefs about exercise is more difficult than it appears and may not give helpful results. Although there is truth to this criticism, use of validated scales has provided useful information that may eventually help to promote appropriate increases in exercise and physical activity levels.

Observational Studies on Body Image and Exercise

Observational studies, which typically compare groups, are usually the first types to emerge in the scientific literature, but there are problems with them. For example, body satisfaction might be compared in two groups of teenagers, those with high and low physical activity levels. Let's say that body satisfaction was found to be higher among those who exercised more. It might therefore be concluded that higher physical activity improves body image. But how do we know whether or not some of the teenagers started

> Observational studies that look at body image and exercise can be prone to error.

out feeling better about their bodies, which *caused* them to be more physically active. Another problem with observational studies is that they often miss elusive, unmeasured factors that might account for the differences that are detected between study groups. In our example, were there questions about socioeconomic status, or whether the students were from schools with mandatory P.E. classes? What if the test was given during summer (when they might be more active) or winter (when they might be under a blanket of snow); would that factor into the answers? Questions that were not asked might account for the disparity between levels of physical activity. Despite such problems, observational studies do provide clues about the connection between insufficient exercise and negative psychological issues.

In an actual 1990 study, the relationship between amount of exercise and body image was observed among 243 college students.[27] The more that the students said they exercised (on a scale from no regular exercise to 10 or more hours per week), the better their body image. This is a good example of a study with results that are not easy to interpret. The researchers, who used the Multidimensional Body Self-Relations Questionnaire and assessed levels of fitness, found that women had to exercise more hours per week to achieve the same level of fitness achieved by men. The researchers speculated that having to exercise more for the same results might account for the higher level of body-image disturbances seen among females.

Physical activity and body image have been studied in pregnant women. This is an interesting, yet complex, group to study because there are dramatic weight changes in a short period of time, and this rapid change in body size and shape may influence body image. One study compared exercising and non-exercising pregnant women[28] and found that the women who exercised had better body images, fewer somatic symptoms, less anxiety, and less insomnia than those who did not exercise. Another study found that women who exercised during pregnancy[29] responded more favorably to changes in their bodies in early pregnancy compared to those who were sedentary.

A 2002 observational study evaluated 410 college students and looked at the relationship between scores on the Social Physique Anxiety Scale and Stage of Exercise.[30] In this study, the higher the level of anxiety about physique, the less likely the students were to be exercising regularly during the preceding six months.

Regardless of the limitations of body image research, most studies conclude that there is a positive correlation between exercising and feeling good about one's body.

Groups at Risk for Insufficient Exercise: Obese and/or Depressed Individuals

As we said in the beginning of this chapter, most Americans do not exercise regularly. This majority is represented by a cross-section of the population, from the young and healthy who may not recognize the importance of exercise to people who think they are too old or disabled to begin. Two distinct groups are particularly prone to inactivity, obese and depressed individuals. Certainly, many obese people are depressed and visa versa; and explanations for the overlap include psychological, sociocultural, neurobiological, and genetic factors.

Overweight and Obese Individuals

Currently, the World Health Organization (WHO) recommends the Body Mass Index (BMI) as the standard for determining weight status. BMI is calculated by dividing weight in kilograms by height in meters squared. Tables are also available to calculate BMI when one's height in feet and weight in pounds is known (www.nhlbisupport.com/bmi/), or it can be derived by dividing weight in pounds by the square of height in inches, then multiplying that result by 704.55.

For example, a 5'10" (70") person weighing 185 pounds would have a BMI of 26.6, as the following calculation shows:

Weight, 185 ÷ Height squared, 4900 (70" x 70") x 704.55 = 26.6.

A BMI between 18.5 and 24.9 is considered the ideal weight range. A BMI below 18.5 is considered underweight, 25.0–29.9 overweight, and above 30 obese. The reason for the division between overweight and obesity is that there are fewer physiological problems associated with overweight than with obesity. Morbid obesity is a BMI over 40. It is called "morbid" obesity because the risk of premature death is so high in this group. Underweight status is also associated with an increase in early death. The more underweight a person becomes the greater the risk of death. Someone with a BMI of under 17.5 would be severely underweight or have anorexia nervosa. However, even though the BMI is routinely used in medicine, it is limited and should not be solely used to determine a person's health.

Someone's weight, height, and BMI are determined by a variety of factors, including (most predominantly) genetics, but also age, gender, diet, and exercise level. While we can control our diet and exercise, genetics—which accounts for about 70% of our weight and shape—is predetermined. Regardless, someone who is overweight or even mildly obese can be healthy with proper diet and exercise. By the same token, being naturally thin is not necessarily an indication of good health.

Unfortunately, being overweight is often used as a reason not to exercise. Carrying extra weight, especially for someone overweight or obese, can make physical activity more difficult; and, one's desire and ability to exercise often decreases as weight increases. Also, excess weight hinders the heart's ability to function well. Not surprisingly, the most obese individuals have the least functional cardiac capacity, and they often have a hard time breathing because of decreased lung volume and less-efficient respiratory muscles.[31] Extra weight also increases the likelihood of developing musculoskeletal and joint problems, such as osteoarthritis. What's more, some obese individuals may not exercise for fear of bringing on a heart attack or stroke. When we add in the fact that large people have a lowered tolerance for heat, exercise can be painful and uncomfortable. It's really no surprise that an overweight person would avoid it.

Extra weight also makes exercise more difficult from a psychological perspective. Many overweight individuals report not exercising because of the shame and embarrassment they feel. They may fear what others might say or think, and will forego exercise because they dread being seen at gyms filled with people who are thinner and more physically fit. Some obese men and women avoid exercising at gyms because they worry that they are too large or heavy to use the equipment. Given the evidence regarding weight discrimination, these fears may be well-founded. Just as we now have exercise facilities exclusively for women to reduce their discomfort of exercising in the presence of men, it would be great if there were facilities designed specifically for those who are overweight and obese. These gyms would include special exercise equipment that might better accommodate these individuals' size, weight, and special needs.

Depressed Individuals

Depression is a very common disorder, which affects approximately 10% of the American population during any one-year period.[32] Ironically, although exercise can help relieve symptoms associated with depression, people who suffer from it are less likely to exercise.

The *Diagnostic and Statistical Manual of Mental Disorders*[33] lists several *mood disorders* (types of depression), which are characterized by some, if not most, of the following characteristics: decreased energy, activity, interest, and motivation, along with low mood, negative thoughts (including thoughts of suicide), social withdrawal, difficulty sleeping, disturbance in appetite or eating, and feelings of hopelessness, helplessness, and worthlessness. The National Institute of Mental Health reports that, in any given year, over 18 million people suffer from a depressive illness.[34] Research also suggests that many patients with Major Depressive Disorder also have a painful physical or medical condition.[35] Given the laundry list of symptoms, we can see why many depressed individuals have little interest in exercising.

Sometimes the depression is so severe that, even if these individuals *could* exercise, they may perceive their initial, less-than-perfect exercise attempts as a failure, or a confirmation that they cannot change or do anything "right." These people might describe their exercise performance as "not enough," or "not good enough," or conclude that, "It doesn't matter." This type of thinking can be carried to such an extreme that planned physical activity actually causes them to feel *more* depressed. By contrast, non-depressed people usually feel better after exercise and view it in a positive way.

Depression can affect eating in two directions. Some overeat to comfort or distract themselves from their inner pain. This increase in eating may *decrease* the likelihood of exercise for many of these individuals because eating seems more enjoyable and is much easier to do. Other depressed individuals may eat less due to a dwindling appetite or simply a decrease in the capacity to enjoy anything, including food. For them, the reduction in energy resulting from eating less also decreases their likelihood of being physically active.

Chronic Illness, Medications, and Insufficient Exercise

People with Chronic Illnesses

The likelihood of chronic illnesses is increased when people are sedentary, but the reverse is true also—people with chronic illnesses are less likely to exercise. For example, heart disease may cause a formerly active person to experience chest pain or shortness of breath and might cause her to decrease her physical activity. Consider Sybil's story.

Until she was about age 50, Sybil enjoyed dancing and often went on weekend trips to participate in dance marathons with friends. Then, she changed jobs, had to drive much farther to work, became more easily fatigued, and had more job-related stress. She had less time and energy for dancing, gained a modest amount of weight, and developed atrial fibrillation (a heart condition in which the heart beats irregularly, with a decrease in the amount of oxygen to the body's tissues). She had to take several different medications to control the atrial fibrillation, most of which are associated with weight gain. Eventually she had heart surgery and multiple complications, but she was able to return to work, albeit more tired and weak than she had been previously. Her physical activity decreased further and her weight increased more and more. Sybil was discouraged and resisted exercising because her capacity was so far diminished from her earlier marathon condition. Nonetheless, she tried to be more physically active, even though she tired easily and sometimes had difficulty climbing the steps to her apartment. However, it's important to note that Sybil worked hard in physical therapy to improve her strength and endurance. But, she could no longer dance as she had previously.

Sybil's story is a good example of the way in which a chronic illness can negatively affect physical activity levels and that illnesses do not have to stop someone from exercising. The emergence of a disease—or injury for that matter—can be an emotional blow to one's sense of self and one's sense of body integrity. It takes time to accept the changes in one's body and to grieve for the loss of physical or emotional health before being able to commit to an exercise regimen, especially when it may be very different from what was possible prior to the development of the illness.

In Chapter Nine, we will further discuss how physical activity can improve the quality of life among individuals with chronic illnesses and explain that disease-related symptoms can be reduced with exercise.

Effects of Chronic Mental Illnesses

Many psychiatric illnesses are associated with decreased physical activity levels. For example, patients with schizophrenia are likely to be less active for several reasons. First, this illness often begins during adolescence or young adulthood and is accompanied by suspiciousness and paranoia; thus, at ages when other people are participating in leisure time sports or other activities, schizophrenics are less likely to join them. Also, they are often prescribed medications that result in sedation, which decreases the likelihood that the person will exercise. Individuals are less likely to exercise if they have agoraphobia (afraid to go outside) or psychotic disorders (often too suspicious to go to health clubs or participate in sports). Also, medications used to treat other serious mental illnesses, such as depression, bipolar disorder, or anxiety disorders can cause sedation, which may result in decreased physical activity and subsequent weight gain.

Medications that Affect Physical Activity

Many medications can cause a decrease in physical activity, promote weight gain, or both. Until the last decade, there was little medical interest in the effect of medications on physical activity or weight. Although the Food and Drug Administration (FDA) requires noting sedation as a side-effect, nothing has to be listed regarding physical activity levels. In addition, until recently, the FDA did not require that studies of medications specifically determine whether or not there were changes in weight during drug trials. Thus, for many older (and less expensive) drugs we have anecdotal and clinical information about this, but few formal research findings.

The categories of medications that can cause weight or physical activity changes are broad. For example, medications for diabetes mellitus, including insulin and rosiglitazone maleate (Avandia), cause weight gain. Physical activity may decline as a result. Another is prednisone, which is commonly prescribed for autoimmune diseases, including rheumatoid arthritis. Both rosiglitazone and prednisone cause weight gain through multiple mechanisms, including an increase in fluid retention and fat stores, and a subsequent decline in spontaneous physical activity. Some medications may also affect metabolic rate in ways that increase weight or decrease activity levels.

As noted previously, psychiatric medications—such as olanzapine, a second-generation antipsychotic used for the treatment of schizophrenia—often cause decreases in both physical activity (via sedative effects) and weight gain. Also, many antidepressants—including mirtazapine (Remeron) and amytriptyline—can cause somnolence (drowsiness) and significant long-term weight gain.[36] When it comes to medications, it is often not clear which comes first: sedation that leads to an increase in weight or weight gain that leads to a decrease in physical activity, or a combination of the two. One thing that is clear is that someone who is fatigued is less likely to exercise.

Notes

1. *fewer than 50% of Americans exercise regularly. Physical Activity Statistics* (2005). Department of Health and Human Services, Centers for Disease Control and Prevention.

2. *are overweight or obese. Prevalence of Overweight and Obesity among Adults. United States, 2003-2004.* Department of Health and Human Services, National Center for Health Statistics.

3. *role physical activity plays in weight maintenance.* In *The Pima Indians: Pathfinders for Health.* National Institutes of Health, National Institute of Diabetes and Digestive and Kidney Diseases, NIH Publication No. 95-3821. Available: www.cdc.gov/nccdphp/dnpa/physical/stats/index.htm.

4. *ethnic groups in the United States.* Gohdes D: Diabetes in North American Indians and Alaska Natives. In *National Diabetes Data Group, Diabetes in America,* 2nd ed. NIH Publication No. 95-1468, pp. 683-701. Bethesda, MD: National Institute of Diabetes and Digestive and Kidney Diseases, National Institutes of Health, 1995.

5. *concept of a "thrifty genotype."* Damcott CM, Sack P, Shuldiner AR: The genetics of obesity. *Endocrinol Metab Clin North Am* 32:761-786, 2003.

6. *genetic factors regulating food intake and voluntary physical activity.* Ravussin E, Bogardus: Energy balance and weight regulation: genetics versus environment. *Br J Nutr 83*:Suppl 1: S17-20, 2000.

7. *report by the Surgeon General (1996).* Physical Activity and Health: A Report of the Surgeon General. Executive Summary. U.S. Department of Health and Human Services, Centers for Disease Control and Prevention, National Center for Chronic Disease Prevention and Health Promotion, The President's Council on Physical Fitness and Sports, 2005.

8. *one study.* Haase A, Steptoe A, Sallis JF, Wardle J: Leisure-time physical activity in university students from 23 countries: associations with health beliefs, risk awareness, and national economic development. *Preventive Medicine 39:*182-190, 2004.

9. *had increased to 65%.* Popkin BM: The shift in stages of the nutrition transition in the developing world differs from past experiences! *Public Health Nutrition 5:* 205-214, 2002.

10. *between 1985 and 2000.* Wu Y: Overweight and obesity in China. *British Medical Journal 333:* 362-363, 2006.

11. *for several reasons.* Popkin BM: Nutrition in transition: the changing global nutrition challenge. *Asia Pacific Journal of Clinical Nutrition 10:* S13-S18, 2001.

12. *on the rise.* Huon GF, Mingyi Q, Oliver K, Xiao G: A large-scale survey of eating disorder symptomatology among female adolescents in the People's Republic of China. *International Journal of Eating Disorders 32:*192-205, 2002.

13. *rate of obesity is a mere 8.8%.* Marques-Vidal P, Ruidavets JB, Amouyel P, Ducimetiere P, Arveiler D, Montaye M, Haas B, Bingham A, Ferrieres J: Change in cardiovascular risk factors in France, 1985-1997. *Eur J Epidemiol 19*:25-32, 2004.

14. *way of life are significant.* Romon M, Duhamel A, Collinet N, Weill J: Influence of social class on time trends in BMI distribution in 5-year-old French children from 1989 to 1999. *Int J Obes Relat Metab Disord 29*:54-59, 2005.

15. *National Center for Health Statistics:* National Center for Health Statistics. (2004). *Health, United States, 2004.* Hyattsville, MD.

16. *less than 120/80 mm Hg.* Chobanian AV, Bakris GL, Black HR, Cushman WC, et al: Seventh report of the joint national committee on prevention, detection, evaluation, and treatment of high blood pressure. *Hypertension 42*:1206-1252, 2003.

17. *we think, see, hear.* Cited by Andreasen N: Available: www.schizophrenia.com/research/adreasen.htm. See also Lloyd G (Ed.): *Hippocratic Writings.* Penguin Books, 1978, p. 248.

18. *influence each other.* Roccatagliata G: Classical Psychopathology. *A Pictoral History of Psychology.* W.G. Bringmann, Ed. Chicago, Ill. Quintessence Publishing, 1997, p. 386.

19. *his classic drawing of pain.* Descartes R. Cited in Carter RB: *Descartes' Medical Philosophy: The Organic Solution to the Mind-Body Problem.* Baltimore, Johns Hopkins University, 1983.

20. *a bodily ego.* In: Freud S: *The Ego and the Id.* WW Norton & Co., New York, 1960.

21. *Figure Rating Scale.* Stunkard A, Sorenson T, Schlusinger F: Use of the Danish Adoption Register for the Study of Obesity and Thinness. In *The Genetics of Neurological and Psychiatric Disorders. S. Key (Ed.),* 1980, p. 119.

22. *Body Parts Satisfaction Scale.* Berscheid E, Walster E, Bohrnstedt G: The happy American body: A survey report. *Psychology Today 7*:119-131, 1973.

23. *Self-Relations Questionnaire.* Cash TF: The Multidimensional Body Self-Relations Questionnaire. Unpublished manual. Department of Psychology, Old Dominion University, Norfolk, Virginia, 1994.

24. *Physique Anxiety Scale.* Hart EA, Leary MR, Rejeski WJ: The measurement of social physical anxiety. *Journal of Sport and Exercise Psychology 11*:94-104, 1989.

25. *Self-Efficacy Scale.* Ryckman R, Robbins MA, Thornton B, Cantrell P: Development and validation of a physical self-efficacy scale. *Journal of Personality and Social Psychology 42*:891-900, 1982.

26. *have argued.* Rhodes RE, Plotnikoff RC, Spence JC: Creating parsimony at the expense of precision? Conceptual and applied issues of aggregating belief-based construction in physical activity research. *Health Educ Res 19*:392-405, 2004.

27. *243 college students.* Adame DD, Johnson TC, Cole SP, Matthiasson H, Abbas MA: Physical fitness in relation to amount of physical exercise, body image, and locus of control among college men and women. *Percept Mot Skills 70:*1347-1350, 1990.

28. *non-exercising pregnant women.* Goodwin A, Astbury J, McMeeken J: Body image and psychological well-being in pregnancy. A comparison of exercisers and non-exercisers. *Aust N Z J Obstet Gynaecol 40:*442-447, 2000.

29. *during pregnancy.* Boscaglia N, Skouteris H, Wertheim EH: Changes in body image satisfaction during pregnancy: a comparison of high exercising and low exercising women. *Aust N Z J Obstet Gynaecol 43:*41-45, 2003.

30. *Stage of Exercise.* Kratzer ME: The relationship between social physique anxiety and stage of exercise behavior change. Master of Education thesis, University of Cincinnati, 2002. Available at http://www.ohiolink.edu.

31. *respiratory muscles.* World Health Association—Nutrition for Health and Development Update Revised 3/3/2004 at www.who.int/nut (retrieved 6/26/2005).

32. *any one-year period.* In: *The Invisible Disease: Depression.* NIH Publication No. 01-4591 www.nimh.nih.gov/publicat/invisible.cfm (retrieved June 26, 2005)

33. *Diagnostic and Statistical Manual of Mental Disorders IV* Text Revision, American Psychiatric Association, 2000.

34. *from a depressive illness:* National Institute of Mental Health. (2000). *Depression.* Available: www.nimh.nih.gov/publicat/depression/cfm (retrieved November 28, 2005).

35. *Physical or medical condition.* Ohayon, M. M., & Schatzberg, A. F. Using chronic pain to predict depressive morbidity in the general population. *Arch Gen Psychiat 60:* 39-47, 2003.

36. *long-term weight gain.* Bremmer JD: A double-blind comparison of Org 3770, amitriptyline and placebo in major depression. *J Clin Psychiatry 56:*519-525, 1995.

CHAPTER 7

Exercise Balance for Everyone

This chapter describes the main types of exercise: aerobic, strength training, flexibility, and balance; and it has recommendations for developing a training schedule. Also included is an important section on strategies for motivation. Whether you are just beginning to exercise or are looking for a more balanced approach, these guidelines will help you develop an individual fitness program that is just right.

The old adage "moderation in all things" is certainly true for exercise. By now you might be wondering just what is the right type and amount of exercise. In addition to this book, this topic appears on the Internet or in magazines and newspapers. It is quickly apparent that a wide variety of regimes exist, with each endorsed by some "expert" or official organization. Our approach is to provide accurate information to synthesize so you can create a suitable program for yourself. The facts we present here are appropriate for everyone, and in further chapters we will offer more specifics based on age and for people with chronic illnesses.

In this chapter, we go into detail with the steps that can be taken toward a safe and moderate routine. First is a brief questionnaire to determine whether or not medical or physical tests are needed before beginning to exercise. Then, we make recommendations for preventing injuries. Next, we get into a substantial description of the four main types of exercise: aerobic, strength (resistance) training, flexibility, and balance. Examples of each type of exercise are given along with suggestions about establishing a moderate training schedule. Finally, we present professional and personal opinions about motivation and success.

Before Beginning an Exercise Program

Although there are several questionnaires available to help determine if you need to see a doctor before beginning an exercise program, we recommend answering the Physical Activity Readiness Questionnaire (PAR-Q)[1] in Table 7.1.

TABLE 7.1. Physical Activity Readiness Questionnaire (PAR-Q) (A questionnaire for people aged 15 to 69)

Regular physical activity is fun and healthy, and increasingly more people are starting to become more active every day. Being more active is very safe for most people. However, some people should check with their doctor before they start becoming much more physically active.

If you are planning to become much more physically active than you are now, start by answering the seven questions in the box below. If you are between the ages of 15 and 69, the PAR-Q will tell you if you should check with your doctor before you start. If you are over 69 years of age, and you are not used to being very active, check with your doctor.

Common sense is your best guide when you answer these questions. Please read the questions carefully and answer each one honestly: check YES or NO.

Physical Activity Readiness Questionnaire (PAR-Q)	YES	NO
Has your doctor ever said that you have a heart condition <u>and</u> that you should only do physical activity recommended by a doctor?		
Do you feel pain in your chest when you do physical activity?		
In the past month, have you had chest pain when you were not doing physical activity?		
Do you lose your balance because of dizziness or do you ever lose consciousness?		
Do you have a bone or joint problem (for example, back, knee, or hip) that could be made worse by a change in your physical activity?		
Is your doctor currently prescribing drugs (for example water pills) for your blood pressure or heart condition?		
Do you know of <u>any other reason</u> why you should not do physical activity?		

If you answered YES to one or more questions:

Talk with your doctor by phone or in person BEFORE you start becoming much more physically active or BEFORE you have a fitness appraisal. Tell your doctor about the PAR-Q and which questions you answered YES.

• You may be able to do any activity you want—as long as you start slowly and build up gradually. Or, you may need to restrict your activities to those which are safe for you. Talk with your doctor about the kinds of activities you wish to participate in and follow his/her advice.

• Find out which community programs are safe and helpful for you.

If you answered NO honestly to <u>all</u> PAR-Q questions, you can be reasonably sure that you can:

    • start becoming much more physically active–begin slowly and build up gradually. This is the safest and easiest way to go.

    • take part in a fitness appraisal–this is an excellent way to determine your basic fitness so that you can plan the best way for you to live actively. It is also highly recommended that you have your blood pressure evaluated. If your reading is over 144/94, talk with your doctor before you start becoming much more physically active.

Delay becoming much more active:

    • if you are not feeling well because of a temporary illness such as a cold or a fever–wait until you feel better; or

    • if you are or may be pregnant–talk to your doctor before you start becoming more active.

Please note:

If your health changes so that you then answer YES to any of the above questions, tell your fitness or health professional. Ask whether you should change your physical activity plan.

Informed Use of the PAR-Q: The Canadian Society for Exercise Physiology, Health Canada, and their agents assume no liability for persons who undertake physical activity, and if in doubt after completing this questionnaire, consult your doctor prior to physical activity. Source: Physical Activity Readiness Questionnaire (PAR-Q) ©2002. Used with permission from the Canadian Society for Exercise Physiology www.csep.ca..

When Not to Exercise

There are some circumstances when you should not exercise:

•   If you have a cold, the flu, or an infection accompanied by a fever, exercise is dangerous.

•   If you develop a swollen or painful muscle or joint, exercise must be stopped to determine the cause.

•   If you experience a new symptom (for example, greater fatigue with the same intensity of exercise), see a primary care physician.

•   If you develop any of the following physical symptoms, such as: dizziness or faintness, nausea, marked or painful shortness of breath, exercise must be stopped immediately.

•   Symptoms such as chest pain or irregular heartbeat should be evaluated by your doctor without delay.

What Exercise Should I Do?

The best exercise is one that will be continued on a regular basis. Ideally, you should combine a variety of physical activities that are enjoyable and convenient. For many people who exercise consistently, working out is one of the high points of the day. For example, Jennie looks forward to her weekly tennis matches and spends four days a week practicing and doing strengthening and conditioning as preparation for playing well. The actual matches are her passion, but she appreciates the other workouts because they make her perform better. Steve also has a lot of fun by playing a sport. He plays in pickup basketball games three days a week, works up a good sweat, and enjoys socializing with the regular group of guys at the gym. On the other hand, Ron Thompson, one of the authors of this book, is a runner. He likes the solitude and opportunity to be alone with his thoughts while exercising. (Ron's personal insights will be offered later in this chapter.) No matter what approach you take, it is always easier to stick to it if you like the type of exercise. If you are a person who has simply never liked physical activity, find the *least* objectionable activity and stick with it for the sake of the benefits to be gained. You will soon discover that an exercise program can be pleasurable.

There are four main types of exercise, and each type should be incorporated into a successful exercise program. *Aerobic* exercise is vigorous physical activity in which the heart and lungs are forced to work harder to provide oxygen to the tissues of the body. This is often called "cardiovascular" or "endurance" exercise. Examples include jogging, running, swimming, brisk walking, and bicycling. *Strength* or resistance training is an anaerobic exercise, which makes your muscles and bones stronger rather than having significant cardiovascular benefits. Weight lifting is one example. *Flexibility* exercises are also anaerobic; they tone your body by stretching muscles and are important in preventing injuries. Stretching during warm-ups reduces the risk of injury. *Balance* exercises are especially important in middle and later life and help the individual maintain control over his or her body, which can decrease the likelihood of falling. Optimally, all four types of exercise should be incorporated into a comprehensive exercise program, and we will examine each in further detail.

The Activity Pyramid shown in Figure 7.1. is similar to the classic Food Pyramid that was introduced to many of us in grade school. It is a visual tool that describes recommended types of, and times for, various physical activities. The lower level emphasizes activities that can be easily incorporated into your day, such as taking the stairs, walking the dog, shopping, gardening, or housecleaning. *Individuals starting out may need to stick to this level until they can gradually build up the endurance and strength for more vigorous activities.* The next level has aerobics, which should be performed for approximately 30 minutes at least three days a week. The pyramid is a reminder to include strength training and flexibility exercises, which should also be part of warm-up and cool-down periods. Finally, it indicates sedentary activities, which include watching television and playing computer games. These should not last longer than 30 minutes at a time.

FIGURE 7.1. Activity Pyramid

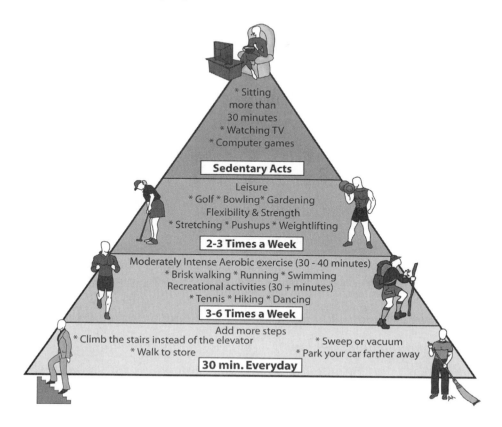

This is a graphic way of understanding recommended physical activity for healthy adults (15 to 69 years of age).

Aerobic Exercise

As explained in Chapter Two, aerobic (cardiovascular) exercise gets the heart pumping faster and increases oxygen consumption. The *frequency, duration,* and *intensity* are key considerations. Generally, after a period of 5–10 minutes of warm-up stretching, most people benefit by gradually building up to at least 30 minutes of continued aerobic exercise. In the younger age groups, and with anyone who is in good condition, the *intensity* should trend toward vigorous activity and the *duration* should be 30–60 minutes per session. For some people it is easier to divide the exercise sessions into two or three bouts of 10–15 minutes at a time. A moderate *frequency* would be three non-consecutive days a week. For a beginner who is obese, even walking will get the heart pounding faster and qualifies as aerobic exercise.

Determining Intensity

There are several ways to determine the intensity of exercise. The simplest is the "talk and sing test." During light-intensity exercise, you are probably able to exercise and sing. If you are only able to talk, then it is moderately intense. If you are exercising energetically, you will not be able to talk or sing.

A more scientific way to assess the intensity of aerobic exercise is by using target heart rates (see Table 7.2). The goal is to increase the heart rate to maximum benefit but without exceeding an age-appropriate level, which is important for avoiding injury. As we age, maximum heart rates decrease; the table takes this into account.

TABLE 7.2. Target Heart Rates by Age

Heartbeats per Minute (% of maximum heart rate)			
AGE	LOW (50%)	HIGH (75%)	MAXIMUM (100%)
20	100 BPM*	150 BPM	200 BPM
25	98	146	195
30	95	143	190
35	93	139	185
40	90	135	180
45	88	131	175
50	85	128	170
55	83	124	165
60	80	120	160
65	78	116	155
70	75	113	150

*bpm = beats per minute

Explanation: Maximum heart rate is determined by subtracting your age from 220. When you begin to exercise, gradually increase the intensity of your exercise to be within the working range of your heart (between 50% and 75% of your maximum heart rate). For example, if you are age 55, over several weeks work toward increasing your pulse rate (heart beats per minute) to at least 83 bpm but less than 124 bpm. We recommend not increasing your heart rate above the high 75% range unless you are a well-conditioned, competitive athlete.

How to Take a Pulse

The way to measure heart rate is to take your pulse for 10 seconds (see Figures 7.2 and 7.3), and then multiply by 6. This will give the number of heart beats per minute (*bpm*). For example, if your pulse is 12 beats for 10 seconds, your heart rate is 72 beats per minute (12 x 6 = 72 bpm).

FIGURE 7.2. & 7.3. Method to Measure Wrist (Radial) Pulse & Method to Measure Neck (Carotid) Pulse

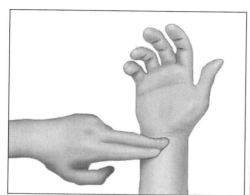 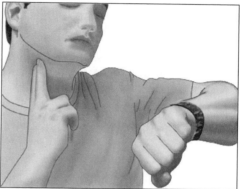

The pulse is the number of heartbeats per minute. Put your index and middle fingers over your wrist or neck as shown. Count the number of beats within a 10-second period and multiply by six.

To determine exercise within target heart rate based upon age, refer to Table 7.2. At age 60, for example, the target heart rate for aerobic activity is between 80 and 120 beats per minute. Note that it is common for heart rate to increase or decrease during an exercise session. Therefore, while learning about your body's tendencies, it is wise to take your pulse every 10 minutes or so to adjust the intensity of activity. If heart rate climbs above target range, slow down. If it drops too low, speed up. You should gradually increase or decrease the frequency, duration, and intensity of exercise. Eventually, you will recognize how hard you are working out without vigilant monitoring.

Another way to measure the intensity of aerobic exercise is by using metabolic equivalents (METs), which is a calculation based on energy expenditure. There is a detailed discussion of METs in Chapter Two. One more method to determine the intensity of aerobic exercise is called the Borg Perceived Exertion Scale, which asks the exerciser to numerically rank feelings of physical stress, effort, and fatigue. This chart can be easily found on several websites. Regardless of the method used to determine intensity, once exercise becomes an ongoing part of your regular routine, you will soon get used to *feeling* what's right.

Weight-Bearing versus Non Weight-Bearing Aerobic Exercise

For people without health problems, an additional recommendation is that at least one day of your regimen include *weight-bearing* aerobics.[2] Weight-bearing exercises work against the force of gravity and keep bones strong and help prevent osteoporosis (brittle bones that break easily). Walking, jogging, hiking, and dancing are excellent examples.

> Healthy individuals should participate in weight-bearing aerobic exercise at least once a week.

People with osteoporosis, knee problems, or other similar concerns need to limit their daily weight-bearing activities. Obviously, activities such as racquetball or fast-moving team sports would be inappropriate. Instead, those individuals are better off with a *non weight-bearing* aerobic exercise, such as swimming or deep water running (with a flotation belt). These kinds of activities put less stress on the body.

Strength Exercises (Resistance Training)

Strength exercises (resistance training or anaerobic exercises) should be performed at least two non-consecutive days per week for a variety of reasons. Strengthening helps to maintain bone density, improve balance, coordination, and mobility, plus it reduces symptoms associated with numerous chronic illnesses. Furthermore, resistance training, in combination with aerobics, may increase your sense of vigor and vitality, improve your mood, and boost your overall sense of well-being.

There are many ways to find a good workout program. Most fitness centers have qualified trainers to guide you throughout the process, there are books and magazines on the topic, and there are a few million entries for "strength-training" on the web. Any of these roads can get you to your desired destination. We recommend basing workouts on the *Growing Stronger*[3] program that was designed by the Centers for Disease Control and Prevention (CDC), which we will soon describe in more detail.

Strengthening programs typically include upper body muscle groups, including chest, back, shoulders, biceps, triceps, sides, and abdominals, and lower body muscles, such as hamstrings, quadriceps, and calves. Some people prefer to work upper and lower body parts on alternating days, but that is not necessary for everyone. Most important, when beginning any strengthening program, start with low weights and fewer repetitions. Very gradually add more weight, additional sets, and more repetitions. Allow your muscles to adjust to the new demands by easing into it. Patience is rewarded, because starting off too aggressively can lead to extreme muscle fatigue, possible injury, and discouragement.

The CDC website provides a wealth of information, including motivation, preparation, staying on track, other resources, and the *Growing Stronger* workout. It is divided into steps, the first of which incorporates a 5-minute walk to warm-up. The initial exercises are intended to improve flexibility, and they include squats, wall pushups, toe stands, and finger marching. The second set includes bicep curls, step-ups, overhead presses, and side hip raises where weights are gradually added. Next are knee extensions and curls, pelvic tilts, and floor back extensions. These are followed by cool-down stretches that help improve flexibility. This set includes carefully and slowly stretching the chest and arms, the hamstrings and calves, the quadriceps, and the neck, upper back, and shoulders. The CDC website has a collection of animations that show how to perform the exercises correctly and safely. *Growing Stronger* is designed for people aged 55 and older, but it is also a good program for any beginning exercisers. Later in the chapter, we present a more vigorous program, with the example of a man who is in his 30s.

Flexibility Exercises

Flexibility exercises (stretching) help develop greater range of motion around the joints. There are two types of flexibility stretches—*dynamic* and *static*. In a dynamic stretch, the muscle is moved through the whole range of motion of the joint, such as arm circles. A static stretch, like a side bend, is when the muscle is lengthened across the joint and held for 10 to 30 seconds. Practicing yoga is a superb way to increase flexibility.

> Practicing yoga is a superb way to increase flexibility.

Although there is controversy over the advantage of stretching in younger age groups,[4] starting young establishes good habits that can be continued throughout one's life. Stretching definitely has proven to be beneficial beginning in middle age because it helps to prevent injuries. It is helpful to do slow stretching exercises for each muscle group, holding each for 10 to 30 seconds. When performing these exercises it is important to stay relaxed and breathe slowly. Stretches can be done alone or as part of a warm up or cool down from endurance exercises. The following flexibility exercises are recommended by the American Academy of Orthopedic Surgeons. Complete this set of exercises twice a week on non-consecutive days to improve your flexibility and ability to stretch. They are adapted from the CDC's "Growing Stronger" website: www.cdc.gov/nccdphp/dnpa/physical/growing_stronger.

FIGURE 7.4. Wall Push-Ups (chest, arms, and shoulders)

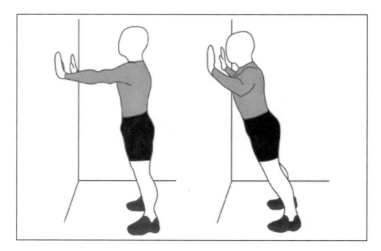

Standing a little further than arm's length away from the wall, place your palms flat against the wall. Slowly, lower your upper body toward the wall while keeping your feet flat. Then, slowly push yourself away until your arms are straight, without locking your elbows. Repeat ten times to stretch and strengthen your chest, arms, and shoulders.

FIGURE 7.5. Knee Stretch

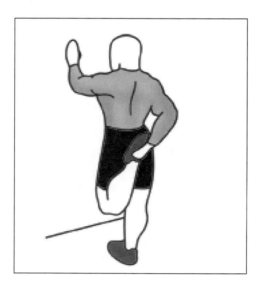

While resting one hand against a wall for balance, grab the top of your left foot with your right hand. Gently pull your heel toward your buttocks and hold that pose for about 30 seconds. Repeat with the other leg.

FIGURE 7.6. Calf Stretch

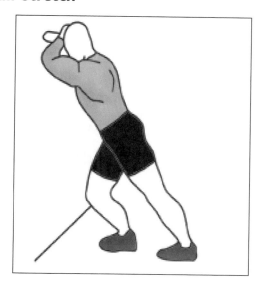

Rest your head on your forearms against a wall. Place one foot forward and the other more than an arm's length away from the wall. Bend your front leg while keeping the back leg straight. Slowly move your hips forward, keep your lower back flat, and allow your calf to stretch for 15 to 30 seconds.

FIGURE 7.7. Lower Back

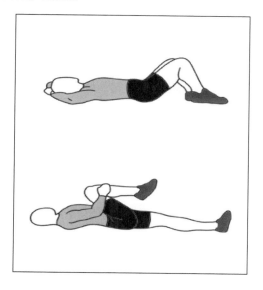

Lie flat on your back with knees bent and feet flat on the ground. Tighten your hip and abdominal muscles at the same time, flattening your lower back. Hold for 5 to 10 seconds and repeat three times. Next, straighten one leg and pull the other knee toward your chest. Try to keep your head on the floor and your back flat. Hold for 30 seconds. Repeat with the other leg.

FIGURE 7.8. Finger Marching

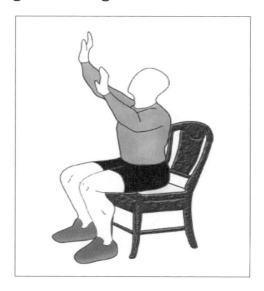

Imagine there is a wall directly in front of you. Slowly walk your fingers up the wall until your arms are above your head. Hold your arms overhead while wiggling your fingers for about 10 seconds, then slowly walk them back down.

FIGURE 7.9. Upper Back Stretch

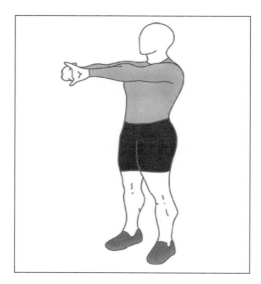

Interlace your fingers in front of your body. Raise your arms so they are parallel to the ground. Rotate your hands so your palms face an imaginary wall. Stand up straight, but curl your shoulders forward. Hold the position for about 10 seconds. The stretch is felt in your upper back and wrists.

FIGURE 7.10. Back and Arm Stretch

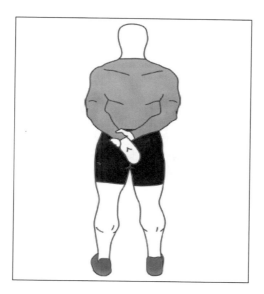

Touch your hands behind your back and reach for your arm just above the wrist. Pull your arm slightly and hold the position for about 10 seconds. Release your arm and then repeat with the other arm. The stretch is felt in your back, arms and chest.

Balance Exercises

Every year in the United States, over 300,000 people fall and break their hips.[5] Balance exercises, especially beginning in middle age, can help prevent this from happening to you. The Mayo Clinic recommends doing a series of balancing techniques at least once daily most days of the week. These are described at the website[6] and include a forward leg lift, forward toe touch, and standing on one leg. Other balancing exercises, such as standing on one foot for 10–20 seconds, walking heel-to-toe, or standing up and sitting down without using your hands can be easily performed during the course of your regular daily life. Tai chi is a perfect activity for maintaining good balance.

Setting Up a Successful Exercise Program

The best programs are convenient and enjoyable, which makes it easier to exercise on a regular and ongoing basis. Your body and mind become conditioned to the routine. For example, Alicia, who was in her mid-30s and worked at a data-processing center was obese, which was creating health problems for her. She ate fast food every day at lunch and simple actions—like getting in and out of the car or going up a flight of stairs—were strenuous for her. A coworker persuaded her to eat quick and healthy brown bag lunches together, and then they'd go for a walk. At first, Alicia struggled to make it once around their office building's grounds; however, before long they circled the block and eventually were taking 20-minute walks around the neighborhood. Alicia's weight, health, and stamina improved, and she developed a deeply meaningful friendship. The lunchtime walks became the high point of her day, and when her coworker was unable to come along, Alicia stuck with the routine out of habit. Although she only does aerobic walking rather than including all four types of exercise, it is still a big improvement over her inactive past.

Find the time to exercise

Try not to think in terms of "all or nothing." Two examples of "all-or-nothing" thinking are: "If I don't exercise for *at least* an hour it won't do any good," and "Unless I exercise *every* day I'm wasting my time." The truth is *any* exercise is better than none. You don't have to exercise for the same amount of time every day, nor do you have to follow the same routine. The first step is to simply become more active in daily tasks. For example, tasks or chores like housework, gardening, lawn mowing, or snow shoveling are all forms of exercise. If there are errands to be run, park farther away from the destination and walk; take the stairs rather than the elevator; bicycle to work or the store.

Nonetheless, as we have emphasized throughout this book, regular, moderate exercise is vital to healthy lifestyle. The amount of time to devote obviously depends on factors such as time or energy, which are unique for everyone. If there is only time to exercise for 10–15 minutes on a particular day, then do that. But if you find yourself too busy to schedule in at least 30 minutes per day on average, you may be over-committed, and need to improve time management skills, or have to learn how to say no.

For many years, I (Ron Thompson) have run every other day for 35–45 minutes, depending on how I feel. I am the first to admit that I do not really like running, but I recognize the importance of exercise and do it. Despite my ambivalence, I am on the road early every other weekday morning. When the weather is bad, I use a treadmill at home and watch television while I run. On alternating days, I use free weights in my garage and go through a 40-minute strengthening routine. I'm a morning person, and when my session is over, I shower, eat breakfast, and leave for work at a time many people are just waking up. Would I like to sleep in an extra hour or so? Sure! But I give up that time for the sake of good health.

Make your exercise convenient

A vital aspect of a successful exercise program is to consider carefully *when* and *where*. I have the most convenient solution by exercising first thing in the morning at or near home. I'm not the kind of person who likes to drive to a gym, pay a membership, and contest with crowds of people vying for the same weight machine. Alicia's lunchtime walking is handy for her. Jennie, the tennis player we mentioned earlier in this chapter, is passionate about her tennis matches, so she's willing to drive to various courts around her city just for the opportunity to play. However, her conditioning is all done locally, including hitting balls against a wall at the local elementary school in the evenings. Women particularly need to feel comfortable in their surroundings; fortunately there are many fitness centers solely for women, or with classes that are gender specific.

Convenience also relates to the specific type of exercise under consideration. For example, running can be done just about anytime and anywhere. It does not require particular equipment or facilities other than running shoes. A lot of people go to fitness clubs or swimming pools close to home or work; and amongst business travelers, it's easy to spot those who are serious about their exercise—they're the ones dripping with sweat in hotel lobbies or alone in the hotels' fitness centers.

A colleague devised a unique strategy to make exercise expedient. She's another person who dislikes running but does it anyway because of the considerable health benefits. Physically, she finds it difficult to run uphill. Psychologically, she much prefers running *toward* her house than away from it. Consequently, her strategy is to have her husband drive and drop her off about a mile from their house by a path without hills. This is a creative and successful way to make her running "easy" because it works for her. Don't be concerned about what others might think. Be creative. Remember, do whatever works for *you*!

Convenience might also involve other people in your life. Take significant others into account when setting up your program. For example, in Ron's case, his wife is *not* a morning person, so she sleeps while he runs. Because he performs his exercise while she is otherwise occupied, they do not miss meals, social events, or anything else they might want to do together. This, in turn, causes his wife to be supportive. Another example is Alicia's, who walks with her coworker and enjoys the benefits of the shared experience.

Make exercise fun

Many people think of exercise as work instead of fun. However, there are many enjoyable physical activities one can pursue: walking, gardening, biking, hiking, skiing, golf, tennis, softball, and volleyball, to name a few. If you're a social person, choose an exercise that involves others to increase your level of enjoyment. Throughout her son's middle school years, Susan spent quality time with him when they'd go to the gym together. Twice a week, they'd be side-by-side on treadmills, sometimes engaged in conversation and otherwise listening to their own headsets and reading their own books; but they were together and it was their way to stay connected during emotionally challenging years.

> If you're a social person, choose an exercise that involves others.

Sports often, by their nature, may require other people. Steve, the basketball player, has been a "gym rat" since high school. He has played on more courts than he can remember and has gotten in games throughout the U.S. and Europe in his travels. He knows which local parks and recreation centers have pickup games and at what times. He shoots baskets in his driveway, practicing various shots and moves; and he follows his favorite NBA and college teams on television and in the newspaper. His lifelong interest in basketball has really been an obsession, but it has served him in a healthy way, allowing him to play well into his 50s.

Individual exercises can be made more pleasurable by listening to favorite music. (On the open road, wearing only one headphone is safest.) Some activities—like walking, running, biking, or rollerblading—can also be made more enjoyable when done in pleasant surroundings, such as a nearby park or beach rather than through your neighborhood. A change in scenery can produce a change in enjoyment. These kinds of exercise can get monotonous, but the boredom can be cured with music, a workout buddy, or varying the routine. Eduardo is another runner with a novel approach. He also runs three days per week. On Mondays, he runs along bike lanes in his neighborhood, choosing different routes. Every Wednesday he can be found on the local junior high school track alternating between timed sprints and cool-down jogs. Then, he rewards himself on Fridays with a leisurely excursion up and down hills in a wilderness area filled with tree-lined paths and a lake.

Another good way a program can be made more fun or interesting is by incorporating different kinds of exercise into your regimen. It not only allows for the development of other muscle groups, additional skills, and social opportunities, it is also another way to prevent boredom. The colleague mentioned earlier who only runs downhill toward home pursues an interesting and broad range of activities. Her program includes hiking, jogging, weight lifting, yoga, and deep-water aerobics. At one point, she was also taking dance classes. Again, be creative and have fun.

Set reasonable and appropriate goals

Reasonable and appropriate means you take into consideration age, health status, and fitness level. For example, running is not an appropriate exercise for someone with painful knees, whereas swimming, deep-water aerobics, or tai chi are better choices. Weight lifting is inappropriate for someone with a bad back; supervised resistance training with exercise machines is better. Some exercisers are motivated by their accomplishments and view an increase (in frequency, duration, and intensity of exercise, as well as different forms of exercise) as such. Nadine started running in her mid-40s and within two years worked her way up to marathons. Peter takes great pride in completing triathlons—he wears his race T-shirts as a badge of honor.

A final thought on setting goals: some individuals stop exercising because they lose motivation when their goals are not quickly realized. If this happens, adjust your goals so they are more reasonable and realistic. A common mistake is to focus exclusively on weight loss. For some people, if they don't lose a specific amount of weight by an exact time, they feel that they have failed despite improved health markers such as decreased blood pressure and lowered cholesterol levels. To avoid such a circumstance, set goals that emphasize cardiovascular endurance, strength, and flexibility.

There are no "magic bullets"

Another mistake many people make in setting up their exercise program involves looking for the "magic bullet" in order to be motivated. Some people believe that once they locate the right gym or the perfect trainer they will suddenly have willpower; but, that's just a setup for failure. Rather than looking externally, find the strength within yourself to keep going. Practically everyone who knows him is aware that Ron is a dedicated runner who religiously sticks to his routine. Friends often ask how he is able to stay committed, and assume that he has great willpower. However, he insists that it has nothing to do with that, but rather he has a way of thinking about exercise that works for him. He exercises because he does not give himself the option not to exercise. Otherwise, he'd probably "exercise that option" because it's a lot easier to do nothing. People admit that this sounds good in theory, but they don't believe they can do it. So he asks them if they will be going to work the next day, to which they invariably reply "yes." How do they know that they are going to work tomorrow? Because they always do. In essence, they do not give themselves the option not to go to work. Even if they wake up and think, "I'd like to skip work today," that's not going to happen. That's how Ron thinks about his running—it is required. For him, exercise is just as important as his job. Make exercise a top priority!

One Sample Workout Program

Mark's story is a perfect illustration of how to start an exercise program at any age. He had just turned 30 and was feeling old, fat, and out-of-shape. While this may seem absurd to older readers, that is exactly how he felt. Happily married and the father of two small children, his life revolved around work and family. The only time he took for himself was to play his guitar now and then on weekends. For his 30th birthday, his wife gave him a membership in a large fitness center a few minutes away from the high school where he taught history, and she encouraged him to give it a try. On the first day at the gym, Mark felt like a fish out of water. Everyone there seemed to be in much better condition than he was, and he was uncomfortable with the whole scene—naked guys walking around in the locker room, a few incredibly muscular behemoths with bulging veins, the rows of attractive women on treadmills who he avoided looking at directly, and the pungent stench of perspiration that had filled his nostrils from the moment he walked in the door. His first impulse was to quickly leave, but instead he fought that instinct and asked at the front desk for someone to show him how to use the equipment.

He got matched up with Sofia, a certified trainer who gave him a tour of the facility, explained how to use some of the equipment, and sent him home with a booklet of standard exercises. That's all he did on the first visit, but when he returned the following day, by appointment, Sofia coached him through an entire series of upper and lower body techniques. He used very light weights with the sole purpose of learning to do each lift correctly, and the trainer suggested that he only do one set at the beginning. By his next visit to the gym, Mark was able to complete a full circuit by himself—again, only doing one set of low weights—and spent five minutes stretching before and after. He continued easing into his routine, working out three or four days per week after school before going home. During the first couple of weeks, he stayed with a single set, but began increasing the resistance so that he had to work just a little bit harder, plus he began using an elliptical cross-training machine. Within six weeks, he had progressed to three sets of a weight that made it difficult to complete the last set and was alternating upper and lower body workouts from day to day.

Now, nearly a decade later, Mark substitutes different exercises in and out of his routine to keep it interesting, but the overall effect has remained consistent. His basic resistance routine includes the following.

Upper Body Workout
(three sets of 8-12 repetitions each)

Chest	Bench press
	Chest press
Shoulder	Overhead press
	Dumbbell lateral raises
Back	Lateral pulldowns
	Seated row
Biceps	Alternate dumbbell curls
Triceps	Overhead dumbbell extensions
Abdominals	Stomach crunches

Lower Body Workout
(three sets of 8-12 repetitions each)

Quadriceps	Squats
	Leg extensions
Hamstrings	Lunges
	Leg curls
Claves	Standing calf raises

Here's His Typical Workout Schedule:

Sunday   Rest

Monday   Stretch (5 min.)
                Treadmill (30 min.)
                Upper body workout (30 min.)
                Stomach crunches (5-10 min.)
                Stretch (5 min.)

Tuesday   Stretch (5 min.)
                Stationary bicycle (30 min.)
                Lower body workout (20-30 min.)
                Stomach crunches (5-10 min.)
                Stretch (5 min.)

Wednesday   Coach son's soccer team at practice (very active)

Thursday   Stretch (5 min.)
                Elliptical cross trainer (30 min.)
                Upper body workout (30 min.)
                Stomach crunches (5-10 min.)
                Stretch (5 min.)

Friday   Stretch (5 min.)
                Stationary bicycle (30 min.)
                Lower body workout (20-30 min.)
                Stomach crunches (5-10 min.)
                Stretch (5 min.)

Saturday   Coach son's soccer team at game (mildly active)

Preventing Injuries

Anyone who exercises regularly is familiar with muscle aches and soreness, but sports injuries have increased in recent years and are most common amongst children and adolescents, older adults, and women of all ages. Researchers are unclear about why women are more vulnerable to injury than men, but the National Collegiate Athletic Association (NCAA)[7], for example, has reported that female basketball and soccer players are six times more likely to suffer injuries to the anterior cruciate ligament (ACL) of the knee than are their male counterparts. Early speculation centered on conditioning and methods of training, but other factors include structural differences of the knee and thigh muscles, hormonal influences, biomechanics (how females jump and twist compared to males), and the loss of bone mass. The rise in injuries amongst people 65 and older is attributed to the fact that people are living longer and more of them are exercising.[8]

Most injuries are not severe and can be prevented. There are several common-sense precautions that can be taken to avoid injury when undertaking an exercise program. The most important recommendation is to *listen to your body*. The well-known saying "no

> The most important recommendation for injury prevention is to listen your body.

pain, no gain" is misleading. Pain is your body's way of warning you that something is wrong. If you're exercising, pain means you should stop immediately and not continue until you or a healthcare professional can determine the nature of the problem and how to remedy it. The recommendations are based on The American Academy of Orthopedic Surgeons and The National Institute of Arthritis and Musculoskeletal and Skin Diseases (NIAMS)[9] for preventing injuries. See Table 7.3. on the next page.

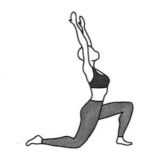

TABLE 7.3. Ten Steps to Preventing Injuries

1. Begin slowly and increase gradually. Follow the 10% rule. That is, increase the intensity or duration of your exercise by 10% or less every week, and do not exceed 75% of your maximum heart rate.

2. Warm up for 5-10 minutes by stretching. This could include walking at a normal pace.

3. Drink about 16 ounces (1/2 liter) of water and consume a moderate amount of food during the two hours before exercise.

4. Be careful not to overexert. Keep the intensity and duration of your exercise within your maximum threshold for exertion.

5. Rest. Try to get six to eight hours of sleep the night before you exercise.

6. If you don't know what exercise to do, ask your doctor or consult with a personal trainer or physical therapist.

7. Dress appropriately. This includes using safety gear and the right kinds of shoes for the activity.

8. If you use exercise equipment, read the instructions carefully and ask for guidance if you are unsure.

9. Try a variety of exercises. It is often helpful to gradually build up to being able to do several different exercises and rotate among these activities. For example, you might alternate jogging, walking, and swimming on successive days.

10. Stop exercising if you develop shortness of breath, pain, light-headedness, chest pain, or irregular, rapid or fluttery heart beat.

Most Important: Listen to Your Body.

Common Musculoskeletal Injuries and Treatment

A number of acute and chronic musculoskeletal injuries can occur with exercise. The most common are muscle sprains, strains, torn ligaments and tendons, dislocated joints, and fractures. A *sprain* is an injury to joint ligaments, which are the bands of tissue that connect one bone to another. A *strain* is damage to the fibers that attach the muscle to the bone.

Can I Treat the Problem at Home?

When musculoskeletal problems develop, it is often difficult to decide whether to seek medical help or manage it at home. NIAMS recommends contacting a physician if you experience *any* of the following symptoms: (1) severe pain, swelling, or numbness; (2) weight on the area is intolerable; or (3) an old injury, which had previously caused a dull ache, begins to swell or the joint becomes unstable. If these symptoms are *not* present, it is usually safe to begin treatment at home. In many instances, over-the-counter pain relief medications, including anti-inflammatory drugs, will be safe and effective. The recommended home treatment follows the PRICE principle:[10]

- **P**rotect the injured muscle or joint from further injury.

- **R**educe or restrict exercise or movement for 48–72 hours.

- **I**ce the injured area 15–20 minutes, 4–8 times a day.*

- **C**ompress the injured area with elastic wraps (do not cut-off blood circulation).

- **E**levate the injured area above the level of the heart to decrease swelling.

* Heat should be avoided immediately after an injury because it can cause internal bleeding or swelling. Apply heat to relieve tension and promote relaxation of the joint or muscle only after the swelling goes down.

This strategy should be used for the first two or three days after suffering the injury, followed by a gradual increase in gentle movements of the muscle or joint, mild strength exercise, and continued ice. Only then should you move to the next stage of rehabilitation, which involves *gradually* resuming usual activities. If pain develops, activities may have been resumed too quickly or intensely. If there is no gradual and continuing improvement, you should consult your doctor.

Notes

1. Physical Activity Readiness Questionnaire (PAR-Q)(revised 2002). Canadian Society for Exercise Physiology. Available: www.cdc.gov/nccdphp/dnpa/physical/growing_stronger.

2. *weight bearing aerobics* Kohrt WM, Bloomfield SA, Little KD, Nelson ME, Yingling VR: American College of Sports Medicine Position Stand: physical activity and bone health. *Med Sci Sport Exerc* 36:1985–1996, 2004.

3. Growing Stronger is available at: www.cdc.gov/nccdphp/dnpa/physical/growing_stronger

4. *stretching in younger age groups.* Andersen JC: Stretching before and after exercise: effect on muscle soreness and injury. *J Ath Train* 40:218–220, 2005.

5. *break their hip.* Wehren LE, Magaziner J: Hip fracture: risk factors and outcomes. *Curr Osteoporosis Rep* 1:78–85, 2003.

6. Mayo Clinic website http://www.mayoclinic.com/health/balance-exercises/SM00049&slide=1.

7. National Collegiate Athletic Association. Report of the NCAA Committee on Women's Athletics (CWA). www.ncaa.org

8. *more of them are exercising.* American Academy of Orthopedic Surgeons. Keep Active-Safe at any Age. Available: www.orthoinfor.aaos.org/brochure.

9. Arthritis and Musculoskeletal and Skin Diseases (NIAMS). Handout on Sports Injuries. Available: www.niams.nih.gov/hi/topics/sports_injuries/SportsInjuries.htm.

10. Price principle. Miller L: Sprains and Strains: What They Are and What to Do About Them. American College of Sports Medicine. Available: www.acsm.org.

CHAPTER 8

Exercise for Different Age Groups

Although exercise is beneficial for almost everyone, the intensity, duration, and type of activity that is most appropriate differs among age groups. In this chapter, we will look at various age groupings based on Erikson's stages of development, the obstacles that each group faces, and practical ways to promote healthy fitness from birth to old age. There is also a section about pregnant and postpartum women.

Before the 1900s, physical labor was such an integral part of the average American's life that a person's activity level was primarily determined by how much work he or she was able to do. Children performed necessary chores on the farm or around the house alongside their parents and even grandparents. The intensity and duration of his or her labor continued to increase until adulthood and was maintained as long as that person was able to work. In contemporary America, however, daily physical tasks have decreased dramatically for all age groups, largely due to modern conveniences.

The problem we now face is how to help a culturally sedentary population to increase activity. In the last decade, the medical community has realized that, in order to achieve this goal, specific strategies are needed for different age groups. Facilitating appropriate physical activity for a preschooler is very different from designing an exercise routine for a post-menopausal woman or an elderly man. We find it convenient to look at these various age groupings by using the stages of development model proposed by Erik Erikson (1902–1994), a well-respected German psychoanalyst and psychologist who was most famous for furthering Freud's ideas on this subject.[1]

Erikson believed that our personalities gradually unfold during eight stages of life and that success or failure at each phase influences the next. Each stage involves mastering two concepts that require balance. For example, the infant's task is "trust" and "mistrust" because he or she need to learn to trust others but not be *too* trusting. If a developmental stage is managed successfully then that person gains a certain psychosocial strength; if not, maladaptations, or poor adjustments, may develop.

Erikson's ideas about the interaction of generations and significant relationships can help us to understand exercise balance. For instance, development during infancy (birth to age one) is significantly influenced by the relationship with one's mother. In contrast, the most important relationships in adolescence (ages 12–18) are with peer groups and role models, while during young adulthood (20s–early 30s) they are primarily with partners and friends (see Table 8.1). Recognizing and understanding each stage of development and its associated relationships help in designing effective exercise programs. Thus, if we want to alter the activity levels of an infant, the relationship with the mother is key, whereas strategies that involve the peer group or role models are more likely to be effective for an adolescent.

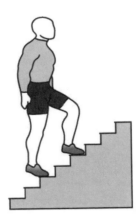

TABLE 8.1. Stages of Psychosocial Development (Erik Erikson)

Stage (age)	Psycho-social crisis	Significant relations	Psychosocial virtues	Maladaptions & malignancies
I. Infant (0-1)	trust vs. mistrust	mother	hope, faith	sensory distortion—withdrawal
II. Toddler (2-3)	autonomy vs. shame & doubt	parents	will, determination	impulsivity—compulsivity
III. Preschooler (3-6)	initiative vs. guilt	family	purpose, courage	ruthlessness—inhibition
IV. School age (7-12)	industry vs. inferiority	neighborhood, school	competence	narrow virtuosity—inertia
V. Adolescence (12-18)	ego-identity vs. role-confusion	peer groups, role models	fidelity, loyalty	fanaticism—repudiation
VI. Young adult (20s-early 30s)	intimacy vs. isolation	partners, friends	love	promiscuity—exclusivity
VII. Middle adult (late 30s-50s)	self-absorption vs. generativity	co-workers, home	care	rejection—overextension
VIII. Older adult (50s and beyond)	despair vs. integrity	"my kind," mankind	wisdom	desperation—presumption

The stages of psychosocial development (as described by Erik Erikson) should be kept in mind when developing strategies to increase physical activity levels at different ages.

In the same way that mastering psychosocial skills helps a person to mature and grow, people who learn exercise habits at a young age move with less effort to the more strenuous fitness activities of adulthood and are most likely to remain physically active throughout their lives. Following Erikson's subdivisions, we can apply general types of exercise to each subgroup.

TABLE 8.2. Exercise Type by Developmental Stage

Age	Stage	Exercise Type
0-1	Infant	Exercise with mother
2-3	Toddler	Exercise with parents; parents model activity
3-6	Preschooler	Family play; childcare center activities
7-12	School age	Physical education, sports
12-18	Adolescence	Sports, peers, multi-component programs; mother-daughter pairs
20s-early 30s	Young adult	After-work team sports; family activities
Late 30s-50	Middle adult	Work place activities; physician input
50s & beyond	Older adult	Group activities; physician's exercise prescription

Throughout the rest of this chapter, we will address exercise balance for each of these groups. However, note that in the years since Erikson's model was developed, life expectancy has increased and so we have taken his model one step further and propose dividing old age into three subgroups: late-middle age (50–64), young-old age (65–74), and old-old age (75+).

Infants, Toddlers, and Preschoolers

Sedentary, overweight, or obese children are liable to become obese adults,[2] and children of inactive parents are likely to be inactive themselves. Both groups have a greater likelihood of developing associated metabolic, psychological, and physical complications. However, on the other hand, active youngsters who continue to exercise throughout adulthood are generally healthier in every way. We believe that overweight and obesity in children and adults are *social* problems[3] that become *medical* problems. Actually, our bodies are responding to a plentiful food supply and reduced activity exactly as we would expect—by storing fat.

Several societal trends have caused a decrease in physical activity in preschoolers. The most obvious difference between rural life of a century ago and today's digital age is the increased "screen time" (e.g., watching television, working at the computer, playing video games), and this is directly related to decreased physical activity, increased consumption of high-calorie, high-fat foods, and a greater likelihood of becoming overweight or obese. Despite the negative health consequences, parents encourage these sedentary activities for a variety of reasons: it is easier to care for children if they're watching TV or playing a video game; early familiarity with computers improves a child's ability to function in our society; and, they may be perceived to be safer in front of a screen than playing outside of the home. For toddlers and other children, having access to safe playgrounds and physical activity programs in childcare centers and schools is too often a luxury instead of the norm.

Another factor that leads to a decrease in preschool physical activity is the tendency of adults to discourage normal wiggling and squirming.[4] There is evidence that this behavior has a genetic basis and contributes to energy expenditure; these movements are hard to quantify but they may decrease the likelihood of becoming overweight or obese.

According to Erikson's model, the task of the infant (age 0–1) is to balance and achieve a sense of *trust* and *mistrust*; toddlers (age 1–3) must develop a sense of *autonomy* as opposed to *doubt*, and preschoolers (age 3–6) learn the difference between *initiative* and *guilt*. Consistent with Erikson's theories about psychosocial development, the most effective strategies for increasing physical activity among babies and preschoolers are focused on the family.[5] For example, parents who teach their infants to swim reinforce the concepts of trust and mistrust while promoting movement and water safety.[6] During the preschool years, parents can help their children to master a balance between initiative and guilt by encouraging active exploration and play without being unnecessarily critical. If this balance is not met, the child may become ruthless or inhibited. Children of parents who engage in regular physical activity are likely to be more active than children of parents who do not. At this age, playing physical games, such as tag, hopscotch, and hide & seek with parents, extended family, and friends promotes developmental mastery and fitness.

In recent years, classes aimed at increasing this bond while facilitating the development of physical activity have been developed, and organized movement programs for toddlers and preschoolers are often more widely available than for older children. The licensing boards for childcare centers in most states mandate physical activity programs for children that are designed for their developmental stage. While the quality of these programs varies widely, excellent classes can usually be found at a local YMCA, Boys and Girls Club, or other centers. Although the class names will differ from place to place, they include the "Wee Workout"[7] program, where parents and children (3 months to 5 years) exercise together in a mini-gym environment; the "Baby Workout" (3 months to just walking), which promotes muscle tone and hand-eye coordination; and "Crazy Bouncin' Babies" and "Happy Hoppin' Tots" (12–24 months), which require attendance by a parent and present the opportunity for toddlers to master the "autonomy vs. shame and doubt" stage of development. Similar programs are available in most cities and teach children at an early age that physical exercise can be fun, social, and a regular event.

School-Age Children

The task of school-age children (ages 6–12) is to balance industry versus inferiority and achieve a sense of competence. Children at this stage begin to feel competent when they are able to master their schoolwork and responsibilities at home. Although these youngsters continue to be influenced by their family, relationships with people in their neighborhood and school begin to be more significant. Unfortunately, too many schools do not place enough importance on exercise.

In 2006, the percentage of elementary schools in the United States that required physical education (PE) classes was 69%, an increase from 50% in 2000. While that is a positive trend, after the 5th grade, the percentage of schools requiring PE decreases dramatically, so that by the 12th grade only 5.4% of schools require any such classes. Furthermore, even though 69% of the primary grades require some PE, the number of schools that require daily PE is even lower. For example, among elementary schools (1st–5th grades), only 8% require daily PE (150 minutes per week). Only 6.4% of middle or junior high schools require the recommended daily physical activity (225 minutes per week). Even more startling, of students enrolled in PE classes, the percentage who exercised or played sports more than 20 minutes during an average class decreased between 2001 and 2003. Many states and districts are only paying lip service to PE. A large majority do not teach from a PE curriculum, have untrained teachers supervising PE, do not require students to take the Physical Fitness Test from the President's Challenge, and do not follow through with "required" instruction. These findings are discouraging, especially because physical education classes at school should be increasing physical activity among this age group.

Not only are these children getting inadequate amounts of exercise in school, they are largely inactive during non-school hours as well. For example, in 2005, only 35.8% students were physically active 60 minutes or more per day five days a week.[9] Another disturbing finding was that girls generally tend to be less physically active than boys.

> Girls begin to become less physically active than boys in elementary school.

Only 27.8% of teenage girls met recommended levels of physical activity compared to 43.8% of teenage boys, a trend that continues through adolescence.[10]

This is also the age at which children begin—and often stop—playing organized sports. Participation in youth baseball, soccer, football, and basketball is a rite of passage for many eight and nine year olds. In many instances, the less coordinated ones become marginalized on their teams and often quit playing after a year or two. By the time they reach the age of 12, usually only the better players are still interested, and often only the most athletically gifted compete after that. Unfortunately, this dynamic often leads children to stop exercising. One antidote to this problem is to encourage children to participate in non-competitive physical activities, such as skateboarding or bicycling with proper safety gear, playing catch with a Frisbee, dancing, brisk walking, and swimming.

For children ages 6–12, the latest recommendation is that they participate in at least 60 minutes of moderate intensity physical activity most days of the week, although daily is preferable.[11] "Moderate intensity" for children of this age means that the activity does not cause hard breathing or sweating. Ideally these activities occur at school, through organized sports, or with family and friends. Because the funding for physical education classes is often the first to be reduced or eliminated during budget cuts, increased advocacy for school-based physical education classes, as well as sports activities, at recreation and park facilities are greatly needed.

Parents need to set an example by being physically active and incorporating exercise into their own daily life, including playing games or exercising with their children. When children are active, praise them and encourage interest in new activities. Find things that both you and your child consider fun so you can be active together. Always be sure that the activities are safe and age-appropriate and that your child uses proper safety equipment (bicycle helmet, soccer shin guards, skateboard elbow and knee pads, etc.). *Never* use exercise as a punishment. For example, if a child is forced to do pushups after misbehaving, he or she may develop negative associations with exercise.

TABLE 8.3. How Parents Can Increase Their Child's Physical Activity

- Decrease time watching television, playing video games, and/or using the computer.

- Model appropriate physical activity for your child.

- Participate in physical games together and suggest physical activities for them to do with their peers.

- Go for walks, hikes, and bike rides with your child.

- Ensure your childcare center has age-appropriate physical activities at least 30-60 minutes per day.

- Tolerate fidgetiness.

- Join in parent-child activities at the local gymnasium, YMCA, or Boys and Girls Clubs.

- Encourage active games like hopscotch, jumping rope, or relay races.

- Support your child's interest in walking or biking to school (if safe).

- Utilize the Children's Activity Pyramid (see Figure 8.1).

Several studies have found that overweight or obese children (particularly girls) feel less competent in doing appropriate weight-bearing exercise than those who are not overweight or obese.[12] Thus, strategies that improve a sense of competence are likely to be helpful. Physical education classes at school and extracurricular age-appropriate sports are likely to be the most effective, particularly if endorsed and facilitated by parents. Because some girls appear to prefer sedentary activities, special strategies may be needed to encourage them.[13] For example, one study found that a planned 12-week physical activity program with mother-daughter pairs (including walking, hopscotch, jumping rope, and dance) resulted in improvement in muscular strength, flexibility and endurance.

Several comprehensive summaries have evaluated the role of physical activity in the prevention of overweight and obesity in children,[5, 3, 11] and general recommendations include:

- reducing sedentary activities to less than 2 hours per day

- restoring physical education to 30 minutes daily 5 days per week

- increasing intramural sports programs

- modifying the local environment in ways that promote physical activity (for example posting prompts to use the stairs rather than elevator)

- educating families and children (by the end of 4th or 5th grade) about the role of physical education

- recognizing the preferential differences between males and females in terms of physical activity

On the following page is the Children's Activity Pyramid,[14] which is a modification of the Adult Activity Pyramid found in Chapter Seven. It provides a visual description of ways that exercise can be incorporated into the life of a school-age child.

FIGURE 8.1. Children's Activity Pyramid

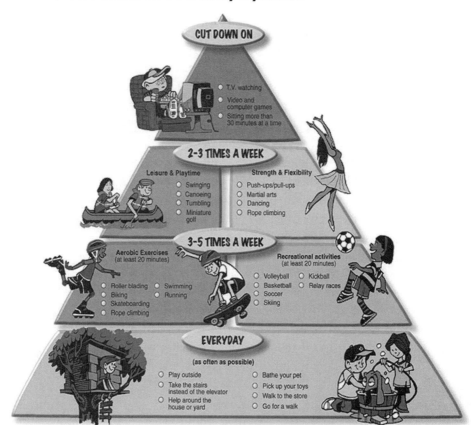

This is visual way to think about the amount of physical activity that is recommended for school age children. The Pyramid was designed by Barbara Willenberg and is available on the web at www.classbrain.com/artread/publish/printer_31.shtml. Copyright 1999, University of Missouri and used with permission.

Adolescents

Somewhere between the ages of 12 and 18, adolescents establish their identity. During this stage, the balance is between *ego-identity* and *ego-confusion* (I am! vs. Who am I?). Successful mastery results in an ability to stay true to one's self and others. During this stage, peer groups and role models are very important and may be more influential in altering an adolescent's behavior than familial relationships, even though the family continues to provide crucial support.

Throughout late adolescence, fewer children meet the recommended levels of physical activity at school. Although the decline is significant for both boys and girls, it is greater for girls, who seem to begin to prefer sedentary activities or are not encouraged to participate in sports. One report found that the majority of girls between the ages of 9–19 engaged in virtually no routine physical activities other than those required by school gym classes.[16] Furthermore, African-American girls were particularly inactive. These and similar findings have prompted new studies of various strategies to encourage and increase the physical activity of adolescent girls, with special emphasis on ethnic groups.

> Parents need to pay attention to the exercise attitudes of their children's friends.

A recent review of seven similar physical activity studies found that among adolescent girls, school-based strategies proved to be the most effective way to increase exercise in girls.[17] There was also evidence that peer-led groups were likely to be successful. One example[18] was an 8th grade peer-led program that encouraged various physical activities outside the usual PE classes. In another study of 10th graders, participants in a 10-lesson, peer-led curriculum exercised an average of 48 minutes more per week than the comparison group. Because peers are so important at this stage, they can provide a negative influence as well. Therefore, parents need to pay attention to the exercise attitudes of their children's friends. A study of 111 families[19] underscores the continuing importance of family relationships in adolescents. The families were first interviewed when the children were in the 5th and 6th grades and again when they were in the 8th and 9th grades. The results indicated that for the girls, their own level of exercise knowledge combined with their mother's physical activity, modeling, and support for exercise predicted their activity level. For the boys, who felt more proficient at exercise, it was the parental model and interest in sports (doing what Dad does) that proved important to their attitude.

The best way to counteract the severe decline in school-based physical education for high school students is to develop positive attitudes and behaviors from an early age. When exercise becomes routine in the elementary or middle school years, the individuals are more likely to continue being active as they get older. However, given the busy schedules that most adolescents endure, the same time-management challenges exist as for adults.

Exercise must be performed on a regular, planned basis, and parents need to persuade their children of its value—that it is necessary for a healthy body and mind.

Young Adults

Young adults in their 20s and early 30s struggle with the conflict between *intimacy* and *isolation* which—if appropriately resolved—leads to love. If not, it can lead to promiscuity or exclusivity. During this phase, activity levels often decrease [20] while relationships with partners and friends are at the forefront. Although this group maintains the level of moderate exercise established during adolescence, the level of *vigorous* exercise decreases dramatically. This fact is particularly ironic because people reach their athletic prime at this age; it is a time when professional athletes thrive. Although some participate in team sports either in college or in after-work leagues, many others take their physical condition for granted.

Only 40% of young adults engage in the recommended levels and about 25% are not active at all.[21] Inactivity is more common among women, and African American and Hispanic adults generally exercise less than Caucasians. The genders differ in a number of factors that influence exercise. Among young women, marriage, pregnancy (see box that follows), raising children, and entering the workforce predicted inactivity.[22] For them, the family is central to social support, whereas men rely more on their friends.

This is the perfect time in life to become active, and opportunities abound. Fitness centers are dominated by this age group, the roads are filled with joggers and bicyclists, and the waters have surfers and rowers. Collegians or young adults in cities can find an array of recreational teams to join, such as basketball, softball, Ultimate Frisbee, hockey, and volleyball. Friends and couples can enhance intimacy by playing sports or working out together. Moderate to vigorous physical activity 30-60 minutes a day at least three (preferably more) days a week is ideal, with strength training two to three days a week to help maintain muscles. The guidelines and "One Sample Workout Program" offered in Chapter Seven are particularly appropriate for individuals in their 20s and 30s.

Pregnancy and Exercise

In general, women who have a low-risk pregnancy and no other health problems can continue to participate in aerobic and strength training exercises.[23] The goal should be to maintain fitness, but not to prepare for an athletic competition. There is evidence that participating in moderate physical activity 30 minutes a day at least three days a week improves the mother's sense of well-being and helps maintain fitness at a time when it typically declines. There are also confirmed medical benefits: the risk of developing gestational diabetes mellitus appears to be reduced by 50% in women who engage in recreational activities during their pregnancies[24] and about a 40% reduction in preeclampsia, which is characterized by elevated blood pressure, swelling (especially in the face and hands), and protein in the urine.

Moderate exercise in pregnant women with no contraindications appears to pose no risk to the fetus, although there is little evidence that it benefits the fetus. Pregnant women should choose exercises that minimize the risk of falls or that might result in abdominal trauma. Scuba diving should be avoided during pregnancy because it puts the developing fetus at increased risk of developing decompression sickness (the "bends"). Pregnant women should consult with their obstetrician for advice regarding exercise.

Postpartum

Although women are often prone to become sedentary after giving birth, there are numerous benefits to exercising. For starters, it helps women return their bodies to a non-pregnant condition. Pelvic-floor exercises may decrease the risk of future urinary incontinence.[25] (Diagrams can be found at your obstetrician's office or on the Continence Foundation website.) Also, there is evidence that regular exercise may decrease the likelihood of postpartum depression.[26] Furthermore, there's a good chance that participating in mother-baby programs will increase the likelihood that the infant will be physically active. One innovative study called "Moms on the Move" incorporates exercise into childcare.[27] Incidentally, moderate activity during lactation does not influence the quantity or composition of breast milk.

Adults

During middle adulthood (late 30s to early 50s), the balance is between *generativity* (nurturing children and being productive in the community) versus *self-absorption*. This stage is successful if the ability to care about others (family, co-workers, society) is developed. If a person does not adjust well, the result is either an overextension of one's self or rejection of the caring role. Important relationships during this phase include the family circle and co-workers.

Because of the responsibilities of middle adulthood, there are many perceived barriers to exercise. These include lack of interest or time, competing demands for leisure activities, and the challenges of balancing the demands of work and home. Some exercisers quit by this age, for example team players who can no longer compete at the same level as younger athletes and those who quit due to injury. Another hurdle is purely physical: the maximum volume of oxygen consumed by the body per minute during exercise (VO_2max) declines by about 9% *per decade* after the age of 25 in healthy but inactive people. However, some research suggests that vigorous exercise may reduce this decline, which can serve as motivation to pursue cardiovascular fitness.

Aerobic exercise in both women and men is key to both preventing and treating cardiovascular disease. As mentioned in Chapter Two, oxygen consumption during exercise is directly related to energy output because it usually increases heart rate. During these adult years, moderate to vigorous physical activity for 30–60 minutes at least three non-consecutive days a week, and preferably most days of the week,[28] is recommended. Additionally, stretching and balancing exercises should be regularly performed at this age.

If someone has not become a regular exerciser by this stage, it may be hard to get started. However, several innovative strategies have been attempted in an effort to bring exercise into the workplace. For example, in the "Los Angeles Lift Off"[29] program, middle-aged sedentary staff (primarily women) engaged in 10-minute bouts of moderate exercise, including low impact aerobic dance and calisthenics, as part of their workday. As health risks increase with age, especially cardiovascular disease, the benefits of exercise become more apparent. The fear of illness is also a powerful motivating force.

Older Adults

People had a shorter life expectancy when Erikson first wrote about developmental stages, so he described only one stage for adults 50 years and over. However, his wife observed an additional stage as Erikson himself aged.[30] As Joan Erikson correctly noted, there are actually *several* important developmental differences among various older age groups. Older age can be divided into three groups: late-middle age (50–64), young-old age (65–74), and old-old age (75 +); and, we postulate that major psychological crises occur at each of these stages, as shown in Table 8.4.

TABLE 8.4. Developmental Stages in Older Adults

Stage	Crisis	Relationships
Late-middle age (50–64 years)	Role model vs. outmoded	Younger colleagues (mentoring)
Young-old age (65–74 years)	Deeper intimacy vs. isolation	Spouse; friends
Old-old age (75 years and beyond)	Appropriate acceptance vs. giving up/acting out	Caretakers (family or professional)

Even this expansion on Erikson's traditional stage model may be insufficient as lifespans continue to increase. In 1990 there were 4 million people in the United States who were age 85 and older—by 2040 it is estimated that there will be 40 million. Just as in every other stage of life, as people age it is important to stay active. Moderate exercise reduces risk factors for heart disease and stroke, and decreases overall early disability and premature mortality. Balance exercises help seniors to avoid dangerous falls. However, the majority of older Americans are inactive. Among adults over the age of 75, 66% do not participate in any physical activity, and 50% have no plans to begin exercising.[31] Only 15% of older women and 30% of older men have continuous activity.

There are several barriers to exercise in these older groups.[32] Among people aged 60–78, the most common one is poor health. Older people may not be able to travel easily to a gym or feel secure on foot away from home. Also, if older people believe their neighborhood is dangerous, they are less likely to walk for exercise than if the surrounding area is considered safe. Another limiting factor is lack of knowledge—they may not realize that exercise can improve health, and may actually view it as dangerous. Many of today's elderly individuals grew up in a time when the need for exercise was not understood or considered valuable. They grew up in an era when physical activity was required to survive and no additional exercise was needed. In fact, some women were taught as children that certain types of exercise were not "ladylike."

A variety of factors increases the likelihood that an older adult will exercise. People who have been active earlier in life may continue or be more willing to start exercising again. A physician's referral after health problems, such as a heart attack, may provide the motivation to join a cardiac rehabilitation class at the local hospital. Sometimes physical activity can be a social outlet in the form of group recreational activities or attendance at a gymnasium. Also, encouragement and praise from family or friends help many people adhere to a program. People who feel confident in their ability to succeed are more likely to participate on a regular and continuing basis, and those who are offered a wide range of choices in terms of physical activities in a safe environment are more likely to participate.

Paradoxically, poor health or the inability to perform daily activities may actually serve as the motivation to begin an exercise program. This may be particularly likely if a primary care physician helps the older person recognize that some of his or her physical complaints might lessen with increased movement (see Table 9.1 in Chapter Nine).[33] A physician can assess an individual's readiness for exercise and prescribe specific advice about how to proceed safely. Elders who work with their doctors in the development of an exercise program often benefit from positive feedback and monitoring.

The key components of a fitness program for older adults should include all four main types: endurance (cardiovascular or aerobic), strength (resistance), flexibility, and balance exercises, which are fully described in Chapter Seven. Although endurance is often central to an exercise program, many older and sedentary individuals initially need to place an emphasis on flexibility, balance, and strengthening.

Summary

The currently available information indicates that activity levels consistently diminish over one's lifespan, even though the benefits of regular physical activity may decrease the likelihood of several chronic illnesses and reduce disability at all ages. The recommendations for appropriate types and times for physical activity for healthy individuals in various age groups are summarized in Table 8.5.

TABLE 8.5. Physical Activity Recommendations: Summary

Group	Time on task
Infants and toddlers	20–30 minutes moderate exercise with parent on a daily basis
Children and adolescents	60 minutes moderate (preferably vigorous) activity most (preferably all) days of the week
Young adults	30–60 minutes vigorous exercise most days of the week
Pregnant women	30 minutes moderate physical activity most days of the week; avoid risk of falling or abdominal trauma; no scuba diving
Breast-feeding women	30 minutes moderate physical activity most days of the week
Middle age adults	30–60 minutes moderate exercise most days of the week; add strength exercises 2–3 days per week
Older adults	30 minutes moderate exercise most days of the week; strength and stretch exercises 2–3 days per week; add balance exercises

Notes

1. *on this subject.* Erikson EH (1980). *Identity and the life cycle.* New York, NY: WW Norton Co.

2. *become obese adults.* Guo SS, Roche AF, Chumlea WC, et al (1994). The predictive value of childhood body mass index values for overweight at age 35. *Am J Clin Nutr 59*:810-819.

3. *social problems.* Matson-Koffman DM, Brownstein JN, Neiner JA, Geaney ML (2005). A site-specific literature review of policy and environmental interventions that promote physical activity and nutrition for cardiovascular health. What works? *American Journal of Health Promotion 19*: 167-193.

4. *wiggling and squirming.* Zurlo F, Ferraro RT, Fonteville AM et al (1992). Spontaneous physical activity and obesity: cross-sectional and longitudinal studies in Pima Indians. *American Journal of Physiology 263*:E296-E300.

5. *focused on the family.* Steinbeck KS (2001). The importance of physical activity in the prevention of overweight and obesity in childhood: a review and an opinion. *Obesity Reviews 2*:117-130.

6. *water safety.* Asher KN, Rivara F, Felix D et al (1995). Water safety training as a potential means of reducing risk of young children's drowning. *Injury Prevention 1*:228-233.

7. *Wee Workout.* Accessed from the internet on 11/2/2005 at www.weeworkout.com/tot

8. *classes was 69%,* Lee S (2007). Physical Education and Physical Activity: Results from the School Health Policies and Programs Study 2006. *Journal of School Health 77*:8. Available: www.ashaweb.org/pdfs/josh77.8leep.435.pdf.

9. *five days a week.* CDC National Center for Chronic Disease Prevention and Health Promotion. YRBSS Health Youth! Youth Online: Comprehensive Results. Available: http://apps.nccd.cdc.gov/yrbss.

10. *continues through adolescence.* ibid.

11. *daily is preferable.* Strong WB, Malina RM, Cameron JR et al (2005). Evidence based physical activity for school-age youth. *Journal of Pediatrics 146:* 732-737.

12. *those who are not.* Fulkerson JA, French SA, Story M et al: Weight-bearing physical activity among girls and mothers: relationships to girls' weight status. *Obesity Research 12*:258-266, 2004.

13. *to encourage them.* Gordon-Larsen P, Griffiths P, Bentley ME (2004). Barriers to physical activity: qualitative data on caregiver-daughter perceptions and practices. *American Journal of Preventive Medicine 27*:218-223, 2004.

14. *Children's Activity Pyramid.* Designed by Barbara Willenberg; www.classbrain.com/artread/publish/printer_31.shtml Copyright 1999, University of Missouri. Used with permission.

15. *school gym classes.* Grunbaum JA, Kann L, Kinchen S et al (2004). Youth Risk Behavior Surveillance-United States-2003. *Mortality and Morbidity Weekly Report 53(SS-2):*1-95.

16. *exercise in girls.* Clemmens D, Hayman LL (2004). Increasing activity to reduce obesity in adolescent girls: a research review. *Journal of Obstetric Gynecol Neonatal Nursing 33:*801-908.

17. *one example.* Kelder S, Perry C, Klepp K (1993). Community-wide youth exercise promotion: Long term outcomes of the Minnesota Heart Health Program and the Class of 1989 Study. *Journal of School Health 63:*218-223.

18. *study of 111 families.* Di Lorezo TM, Stucky-Ropp RC, VanderWal JS, Gotham HJ (1998). Determinants of exercise among children. II. A longitudinal analysis. *Preventive Medicine 27:*470-477.

19. *activity levels often decrease.* A Report of the Surgeon General: Physical Activity and Health. Adolescents and Young Adults. Center for Disease Control and Prevention. Available: http://www.cdc.gov.

20. *are not active at all.* A Report of the Surgeon General: Physical Activity and Health. Adults. Center for Disease Control and Prevention. Available: http://www.cdc.gov.

21. *workforce predicted inactivity.* Brown WJ, Trust SG (2003). Life transitions and changing physical activity patterns in young women. *Am J Prev Med 25:*140-143.

22. *strength training exercises.* American College of Obstetricians and Gynecologists (2003). Exercise during pregnancy and the postpartum period. *Clin Obstet Gynecology 46:*496-499.

23. *during their pregnancy.* Wolfe LA, Weissgerber TL (2003). Clinical physiology of exercise in pregnancy: a literature review. *J Obstet Gynaecol Can 25:*473-483.

24. *future urinary incontinence.* Harvey MA (2003). Pelvic floor exercises during and after pregnancy: a systematic review of their role in preventing pelvic floor dysfunction. *J Obstet Gynaecol Can 25:*451-453.

25. *postpartum depression.* Armstrong K, Edwards H (2004). The effectiveness of a pram-walking exercise programme in reducing depressive symptomatology for postnatal women. *Int J Nurs Pract 10:*177-194.

26. *exercise into childcare.* Fahrenwald NL, Atwood JR, Walker SN et al (2004). A randomized pilot test of "Moms on the Move"; a physical activity intervention for WIC mothers. *Ann Behav Med 27:*82-89.

27. *most days of the week.* Physical Activity and Health. A Report of the Surgeon General. Executive Summary (1996). Available: http://cdc.gov/nccdphp/sgr/summary.htm

28. *Los Angeles Lift Off.* Yancey AK, McCarthy WJ, Taylor WC (2004). The Los Angeles Lift Off: A sociocultural environmental change intervention to integrate physical activity into the workplace. *Preventive Medicine 38:*843-856.

29.   *Erikson himself aged.* Erickson E, Erikson J (1997). *The Life Cycle Completed.* W.W. Norton & Co., New York, N.Y.

30.   *no plans to begin exercising.* U.S. Department of Health and Human Services, Physical Activity and Health. A Report of the Surgeon General. Executive Summary (1996). Available: http://cdc.gov/nccdphp/sgr/summary.htm

31.   *in these older groups.* Schutzer KA, Graves BS (2004). Barriers and motivations to exercise in older adults. *Preventive Medicine 39*:1056-1061.

32.   *increased movement.* Cress ME, Buchner DM, Prohaska T et al (2005). Best practices for physical activity programs and behavior counseling in older adults populations. *Journal of Aging and Physical Activity 134*:61-74.

CHAPTER 9

Exercise for People with Chronic Illness

In this chapter we discuss the almost universal finding that well-planned, moderate exercise helps reduce the symptoms of many chronic illnesses, including those of diabetes mellitus, hypertension, heart disease, osteoarthritis, obesity, and severe mental disorders. We provide recommendations for appropriate exercise levels and outline the benefits. People with chronic illnesses should always consult their physician prior to beginning an exercise program, and at the end of the chapter we look at the role of physicians.

Physical Activity: Benefits vs. Risks

Although the pros of physical activity usually outweigh the cons, it is important to use caution when it comes to people who are chronically ill. Benefits include alleviation of many symptoms, like reduced fatigue in patients with heart disease, the prevention or delay of illness, such as diabetes mellitus or hypertension, and avoidance of some of the effects of aging, such as loss of muscle strength and endurance.

Although the benefits are impressive, the risks are also significant and include the possibility of injury to muscles and bones, sudden cardiac arrest or death, dehydration, heat stroke, and oxidative stress (the accumulation of destructive molecules called free radicals).

TABLE 9.1. Health Benefits of Regular Physical Activity

Health Issue	Benefits and Physical Activity
Cardiovascular health	Improves myocardial performance
	Improves peak diastolic filling
	Increases heart muscle contractility
	Reduces premature ventricular contractions
	Improves blood lipid profile
	Increases aerobic capacity
	Reduces systolic blood pressure
	Improves diastolic blood pressure
	Improves endurance
	Improves muscle capillary blood flow
Body composition	Decreases abdominal adipose tissue
	Increases muscle mass
Metabolism	Increases total energy expenditure
	Improves protein synthesis rate and amino acid uptake into the skeletal muscle
	Reduces low-density lipoproteins
	Reduces triglycerides
	Increases high-density lipoproteins
	Increases glucose tolerance
Bone health	Slows decline in bone mineral density
	Increases total body calcium and nitrogen
Psychological well-being	Improves perceived well-being and happiness
	Decreases levels of stress-related hormones
	Improves attention span
	Improves cognitive processing speed
	Increases slow wave and rapid eye movement sleep
Muscle weakness and Functional capacity	Reduces risk of musculoskeletal disability
	Improves strength and flexibility
	Reduces risk of falls
	Improves dynamic balance
	Improves physical functional performance

FIGURE 9.1. Benefits and Risks of Physical Activity

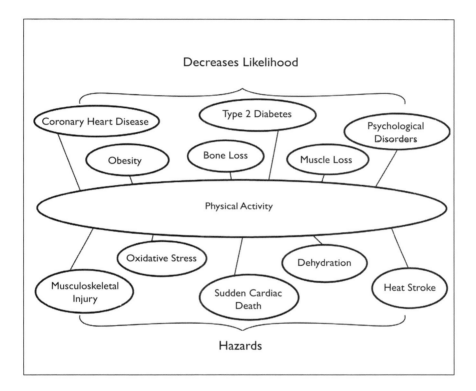

The benefits of physical activity usually outweigh the risks. The possibility of sudden death is rare and the likelihood of it happening can be greatly decreased if you consult with a primary care physician prior to undertaking an exercise program. Adapted from Melzer et al, Physical Activity: The Health Benefits Outweigh the Risks. Current Opinion in *Clinical Nutrition and Metabloic* Care 7:641-647, 2004. Used with permission.

Physical Activity and Quality of Life

Although exercise is routinely recommended both to prevent and treat many chronic illnesses, the actual improvements can be difficult to assess. In the medical world, the term "quality of life" is used to try to determine whether or not various prevention efforts or treatments are worthwhile. In most studies, there are usually ways to measure quality of life: level of pep and energy; ability to carry out routine, daily activities; ability to enjoy friends and socialize, and freedom from symptoms of depression. There are also health-specific quality of life measures. For example, in patients with diabetes mellitus an increased quality of life might include the absence of hypoglycemic (low blood sugar) attacks or a decrease in leg pain caused by peripheral neuropathies.

Physical training among chronically ill patients seems to improve the general quality of life, including improved pep and energy and enhanced functional capacity (for example, the ability to get out of a chair, walk, or carry various items). There is also preliminary evidence that exercise improves mood, irrespective of the underlying chronic illness.

Consult Your Physician

If you have a chronic mental or physical illness, it is particularly important to talk with a primary care physician about what physical activity would be best. It is also likely that a doctor will want to monitor your progress once exercise is begun. Some people may also need an assessment by a specialist, such as a cardiologist. Ongoing consultations may be needed, because many chronic illnesses wax and wane over time. Exercise that is helpful at one time may be detrimental at another.

Do I Need a Physical Therapist?

In addition to suggesting a particular type of exercise, your doctor may refer you to a trained and licensed physical therapist to help restore function, improve mobility, relieve pain, and prevent or limit permanent physical disabilities. Although there is the option to see a physical therapist without first consulting with your doctor, it is best to work in collaboration. That way, a physician can provide a complete medical history and be aware of the specifics of your exercise program. This is valuable because some illnesses result in particular physical limitations. For example, the inability to move a particular part of the body is often the outcome of a stroke, and a physical therapist can focus on helping a patient regain as much function as possible. On the other hand, a heart attack survivor may benefit from a controlled aerobic workout. Most physical therapists are educated about chronic illnesses and the proper approaches to exercise for sufferers.

Working with a Personal Trainer

In what is a rapidly evolving field, the best current guidance about personal trainers is available from the American College of Sports Medicine (ACSM). At their website, www.acsm.org, an ACSM Certified Personal Trainer is described as "…a fitness professional involved in developing and implementing an individualized approach to exercise leadership in healthy populations and/or those with medical clearance to exercise." The minimum requirements to test for certification are a high school diploma or equivalent and a current Adult CPR (cardiopulmonary resuscitation) certificate. Although the ACSM also recommends several health-related competencies (including a course on appropriate exercises for people with various chronic illnesses), they are not required. However, new levels of training are underway, such as programs for health/fitness instructors, exercise specialists, and clinical exercise physiologists. Fortunately, this will eventually lead to improved and personalized rehabilitation by competent professionals.

Unfortunately, not all physical trainers are well prepared to guide individuals with chronic illnesses. For example, even the ACSM's use of the term "medical clearance" is vague and does not specify what the person is cleared to do. So, it is important to find out from a qualified physician exactly which physical activities are safe to pursue.

Although there are no hard and fast rules, Table 9.2 lists some common-sense guidelines for choosing a qualified trainer.

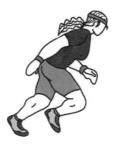

TABLE 9.2. Selecting a Personal Trainer

Facts to Know

1. What are your diagnoses?

2. What are your current medications? How do they affect your ability to be physically active?

3. What are your actual physical limitations?

4. What does your physician specifically recommend in terms of exercise? (Ask for an "exercise prescription.")

5. Does your primary care physician recommend you see a personal trainer?

Characteristics of the Personal Trainer

1. Is the personal trainer certified by the American College of Sports Medicine?

2. Does the trainer understand your physical limitation?

3. Will the trainer consult with your doctor?

4. Does the trainer want to help you devise a graduated exercise plan?

5. Do you feel you will be able to develop a rapport with the trainer?

6. Is the price reasonable?

Many common illnesses occur simultaneously. For example, many people with diabetes mellitus also have high blood pressure. You need to tell the trainer about current medications and how they affect your ability to be physically active. For example, some may cause sedation at certain times of day, so it may be necessary to schedule exercise for times when you are fully awake. Ask your doctor to write an exercise prescription for the personal trainer to use as a guide. It should include your diagnoses, goals, and specific instructions for the type and intensity of physical activity. Also, some personal trainers may encourage the purchase of dietary supplements. Always consult with your physician prior to the use of any food supplement, especially if you have a serious or chronic medical condition.

A Patient Example

Jim was a 61-year-old man who fought prostate cancer for six years before developing metastases and being told that he probably only had a couple of years to live. He also had osteoarthritis in his right shoulder and left knee, which he injured playing college football. After hearing that the cancer had spread, Jim became depressed, gained significant weight (due in part to his medications), and developed high blood pressure. He was told by one doctor to lose weight, even though Jim's situation made that unlikely and ill-advised, given his short life expectancy and concerns about weight loss for individuals with cancer. Nonetheless, he signed up at a local fitness center and began working with a personal trainer on a very intense exercise program aimed at weight loss. The trainer sold him various supplements and did not take into account his medications or college injuries. Subsequently he developed more pain in his joints and began to feel ill.

When he was referred to Dr. Powers, one of the authors of this book, she got him to refocus his goal to gaining muscle strength, vitality, and flexibility. She changed his depression medication from sertraline (Zoloft) to escitalopram (Lexapro), which doesn't cause weight gain, and he stopped taking the trainer's supplements. In fact, he stopped going to that gym, and Dr. Powers referred him to a physical therapist with a specific exercise prescription designed to increase his physical activity gradually and taking into account his sensitive joints. Jim formed a positive relationship with the physical therapist and altered his work schedule in order to attend physical therapy regularly. His energy and mood began to improve even though he did not lose weight. When this book was written, three years after his fatal prognosis, Jim was not only still alive, but he had increased energy and strength and a much better quality of life.

Diabetes Mellitus and Exercise

One problem in understanding the benefits of exercise is that many chronic illnesses are progressive, or tend to worsen. For example, Type 2 diabetes mellitus causes abnormalities in both the action of insulin (insulin resistance) and its secretion (resulting in a deficiency). Over time, even with appropriate treatment and lifestyle modifications, the deficiency usually worsens, and many people end up needing injections. In this case, the benefit of exercise may mean that there is no worsening of the diabetes mellitus or that it is slowed down. By incorporating exercise into one's lifestyle the onset of complications of diabetes may be delayed. These complications include blindness, heart attack, stroke, high blood pressure, and infection.

For diabetics, some of the disease-specific precautions needed before undertaking an exercise program are listed in Table 9.3, which you should review with your physician.

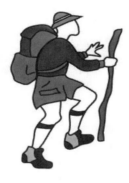

TABLE 9.3. Exercise for the Diabetic: Precautions

General

1. Consult with your physician before beginning a new exercise program; specialist evaluation and testing may be needed.

2. Start and increase your physical activity slowly.

3. Focus on the frequency and duration of exercise over the course of weeks, and very gradually increase the intensity.

Specific Precautions

1. Exercise usually lowers blood sugar: adjustment of medications and carbohydrate intake may be necessary.

2. High blood sugar (hyperglycemia) can be worsened by intense exercise. Monitor your levels.

3. People with associated complications and additional risks should follow these guidelines.

   a. Heart disease: Cardiac assessment and monitoring are required with specific exercise prescriptions to avoid arrhythmias (irregularities of the heart beat).

   b. Peripheral neuropathy (abnormalities of the peripheral nerves that decrease sensation): Be sure to wear proper footwear and conduct regular inspections of your legs and feet.

   c. Diabetic kidney disease: Avoid activities that cause systolic blood pressure to rise above 180-200 mm Hg. This includes some resistance (strength) exercises.

   d. Diabetic retinopathy (changes in the retina of the eye): Avoid activities that increase pressure in the eye, including very resistance (strength) exercise.

Foremost, it is important to avoid either low or high blood sugar (hypo- and hyperglycemia, respectively). Most people with Type 2 diabetes mellitus who participate in mild to moderate exercise of up to 30 minutes per session are not at great risk for low blood sugar unless they are taking insulin or sulfonyurea oral medications. Nonetheless, you should monitor your blood glucose level when first beginning an exercise program to determine whether or not a change in medications is indicated. Also, testing blood glucose before and after a typical exercise period will help detect any changes that occur from exercise.

Even though exercise should be approached with caution, there is evidence that diabetics who engage in regular mild to moderate physical activity experience a decrease in blood glucose—although this improvement disappears within 72 hours. Therefore, the reduction in blood glucose is associated not with overall fitness but with the last round of exercise.[1] Therefore, recurring physical activity is required to maintain healthy blood sugar levels. Paradoxically, strenuous physical exercise can cause an increase in blood sugar, so moderation is usually necessary.

Improved glucose control is associated with a decreased likelihood of heart disease and stroke. Physical activity or exercise also has a beneficial effect in lowering blood pressure in over half of people with diabetes mellitus.[2] If you are over the age of 35 or have heart problems, a heart stress test can be used to determine if the target heart rate during exercise should be lower than indicated on standard tables.

If there is nerve damage in your feet from diabetes (peripheral neuropathy) and you cannot tell if there is pain in your feet while exercising, you may need to take special precautions when undertaking weight-bearing aerobic exercise (such as power walking or jogging). A complete list of diabetic complications and their management is beyond the scope of this book but are described in detail elsewhere.[3] Ask your physician for more information.

Many people with Type 2 diabetes mellitus cannot easily lose weight just by working out. It would take years of nearly daily exercise at moderate intensity to improve their body weight and composition[4]—a level of exercise that is unlikely to be achieved by most people. It is important to guard against unrealistic expectations (especially for weight loss) and to set goals that focus on improvement of glucose control and a reduction in risk factors for heart disease, strokes, or blindness.

A summary of the physical activity program recommended by the ACSM for individuals with diabetes mellitus without significant complications or physical limitations[5] can be found in Table 9.4. The goals include appropriate endurance and resistance training from three to five physical activity sessions per week, involving mild- to moderate-intensity exercise, and developing a resistance training program (strength training program) to improve muscle strength and endurance and to improve body composition. Ideally, resistance training is practiced two days per week with a minimum of 8–10 different exercises that involve the major muscle groups and sets of 10–12 repetitions.[6]

TABLE 9.4. Diabetes Mellitus: Exercise Recommendations

For people who have diabetes mellitus with no significant complications, the following guidelines are recommended after evaluation by a primary care physician. Focus first on the number of times of exercise per week and the length of each session, and then on gradually increasing the intensity of the exercise.

1. Cardiovascular exercise: Perform low- to moderate-intensity aerobic exercise for 30 minutes per workout for 3–5 nonconsecutive days a week. A brisk, half-hour walk is ideal.

2. Resistance training (strength exercises): Do 8–10 exercises involving major muscle groups with a minimum of 10–15 repetitions per set twice a week. See Chapter Seven for more information.

High Blood Pressure and Exercise

About 58.4 million people in the United States—roughly 28% of the adult population—suffer from hypertension (high blood pressure).[7] This illness is associated with an increased likelihood of death from any cause and is part of the metabolic syndrome, which includes central obesity (an increase in fat accumulation around the waist area), insulin resistance, and elevated lipid levels (cholesterol and triglycerides). There is also evidence that more children and adolescents are developing this disorder due to increasing levels of obesity related to decreased exercise and the availability of tasty, high-fat foods.[8]

Hypertension is determined by having blood pressure taken (see Chapter Six). A healthy reading for an average adult is below 120/80 mm Hg. Systolic blood pressure (the first number in a blood pressure reading) increases throughout life and is associated with stiffening of the arteries (arteriosclerosis). Diastolic blood pressure (the second number) increases until the 60s, reaches a plateau, and then decreases. This results in an increase in pulse pressure, which is the difference between systolic and diastolic blood pressure. Increases in pulse pressure are associated with a greater risk of heart disease.[9] Attempts have been made to predict the future development of hypertension in people who currently have normal blood pressure. Several factors have been identified, including a family history of hypertension, an elevated body mass index, a sedentary lifestyle, and an exaggerated diastolic blood pressure response to exercise.[10]

It was once thought that an elevated diastolic blood pressure was more dangerous than an elevated systolic pressure. We now know that both are dangerous. Furthermore, even what was once thought to be high normal blood pressures (systolic between 130–139 mm Hg and diastolic between 85–89 mm Hg) are now defined as "pre-hypertension" and contribute to the risk of heart attacks and strokes.[11] Currently, lifestyle changes[12] (moderation of diet and addition of exercise) are recommended if blood pressure is in the "pre-hypertension range." If blood pressure is between 140–159 mm Hg systolic or 90–99 mm Hg diastolic, lifestyle changes can be attempted for one year, and drug therapy should begin if measurable improvement is not seen within that time frame. That is not to say lifestyle changes should be abandoned if drug therapy begins: blood pressure above this level should be treated with drugs *and* lifestyle modification.

Benefits of Exercise in Hypertensive Individuals

Several types of exercise have been tried and evaluated in patients with high blood pressure, including aerobic exercise and resistance (strength) training. Regular mild to moderate aerobic exercise (walking, jogging, running)—30–60 minutes a day at least three days per week—usually causes some decrease for people with normal blood pressure, but the reductions are greater for those with hypertension.[13] Decreases due to aerobic exercise have been shown to range from 3.4–4.7 mm Hg for systolic and from 2.4–3.1 mm Hg for diastolic. The differences are small, but significant. For example, it has been estimated that a reduction of 3 mm Hg systolic in the average adult population would decrease coronary heart disease by 5–9%, stroke by 8–14%, and all-cause mortality (defined as "death from any cause") by 4%.[14] Vigorous aerobic exercise has been shown to decrease blood pressure for up to 22 hours after exercising.[15]

> If you have high blood pressure, ask your doctor for an exercise stress test before beginning a vigorous workout program.

Resistance training includes both concentric and eccentric exercise. Concentric contraction occurs when a muscle shortens in length and develops tension (for example, the upward movement of a dumbbell in a biceps curl). Eccentric contraction involves the development of tension while a muscle is being lengthened (for example, the downward movement of a dumbbell in a biceps curl). Both types of exercise reduce blood pressure in people with either normal or elevated blood pressure. The range of improvements is similar to that of regular aerobic exercise.

Age, gender, and ethnicity[16] are also factors in the effect of exercise on blood pressure. Studies show that the benefit of moderate aerobic exercise appears to be similar in both healthy younger and older adults. However, children and adolescents with hypertension may not experience the same benefits, and further studies in this area are needed.[17] Although the evidence is limited, women appear to benefit from endurance exercise as much as men. There are also significant ethnic differences. For example, African-Americans tend to develop hypertension earlier and more frequently than Caucasians and have more cardiac complications. The benefit of exercise in African-Americans is not well understood and needs to be further studied.

Risks of Exercise in Individuals with Hypertension

Although mild to moderate exercise (like walking and jogging) among individuals with hypertension decreases the risk of cardiovascular disease, vigorous exercise may actually increase the risk. Strenuous exercise can result in an increased need for oxygen by the heart, as well as a shortening of the time to fill the heart with oxygen, resulting in an irregular heart beat, heart attack,[18] or possibly sudden death.[19] People with hypertension should be evaluated by their physician and undergo medically monitored exercise.

Exercise Recommendations

People with hypertension are urged to exercise, but at mild to moderate (rather than vigorous) levels. A way of thinking about this is called the FITT Principle,[20] an acronym for Frequency, Intensity, Time, and Type.

Although exercising at a frequency of 3–5 days per week is effective in lowering blood pressure, there is evidence that a daily routine is more effective. Since the positive effects of moderate exercise only last up to 22 hours, daily exercise may provide the most benefit. If you're just beginning, start at 2–3 days a week and increase gradually.

The intensity of physical activity should also be mild to moderate to lower blood pressure, such as brisk walking with fairly heavy breathing. If you have high blood pressure, do not perform vigorous exercise until you have consulted with your physician.

The time required to achieve benefits is at least 30 minutes of continuous or intermittent exercise. Dividing the 30 minutes into three periods of 10 minutes each during the day (intermittent exercise) appears to be as effective as continuous exercise.[21]

Aerobic activities supplemented by resistance training are the most effective types of physical activities. Many studies have evaluated endurance exercises—including running, skiing, or swimming—and it has been proven that any activity that uses large muscle groups, is maintained continuously, is rhythmic, and aerobic can be beneficial.

Heart Disease and Physical Activity

Heart disease continues to be a leading cause of death among Americans.[22] The most common problem is coronary artery disease (obstruction caused by atherosclerosis), which can result in chest pain (angina pectoris) or a heart attack (myocardial infarction), where part of the heart muscle dies. If this disease worsens, it can result in heart failure, which means the heart can't pump enough blood to the body's organs and tissues. A person with coronary artery disease may develop shortness of breath, retain fluids, and/or feel fatigued. Regular exercise has been shown to be helpful in reducing these symptoms and may also actually reverse some of the causes of heart disease (for example, increasing the diameter of blood vessels), although most studies have not continued long enough to fully confirm this notion. Nonetheless, exercise that decreases chest pain, shortness of breath, or fatigue does improve a person's quality of life.

Exercise and Heart Function

People with coronary artery disease experience a decrease in oxygen uptake, which may cause exercise to be difficult. Additionally, some treatment medications (including beta-blockers) can negatively affect exercise tolerance.[23] Specialized training programs can gradually increase oxygen uptake to improve the ability of the heart to deliver oxygen to the tissues, which can make physical activity easier.

> Exercise training after a heart attack can improve cholesterol levels, which decreases the risk of a second heart attack.

In patients with true angina pectoris (pain caused by an inadequate supply of blood to the heart), chest pain typically begins when an exerciser reaches a particular heart rate. Regular training results in a decrease in heart rate at the same activity level, which means that the person can exercise longer at the same activity before chest pains begin.[24] In fact, with proper training, chest pain disappears completely in some patients and results in an improved quality of life and ability to function.

A myocardial infarction (heart attack) is a momentary insufficient blood supply to the heart, which results in the death of some tissue. Several studies have found that regular training results in decreases in total cholesterol, LDL-cholesterol, and triglycerides, and an increase in HDL-cholesterol.[25]

Heart failure is a chronic condition in which the heart gets weaker (often, but not always, because of coronary artery disease) and not enough blood is pumped throughout the body. This usually results in an enlarged heart and causes shortness of breath, fatigue, swelling of the ankles, and a decrease in exercise tolerance. There is evidence that gradual training can improve these complaints.

Evaluation Prior to Beginning Exercise

If you have heart disease of any kind, it is imperative that before undertaking an exercise program you consult with your physician. You will probably be given a graded exercise stress test supervised by a cardiologist, who can then recommend the safest type of physical activity. Afterwards, a primary care physician should monitor your condition and progress as you gradually increase exercise frequency, intensity, and duration.

Most people who have had a heart attack are encouraged to enter a cardiac rehabilitation program. The first two weeks are usually confined to brief stints of walking, often under medical supervision. As strength and endurance improve, supervision can be less constant unless one is at particular risk, which can be determined by a stress test. Irregular heart rhythms (arrhythmias) developed during the stress test may require special limitations to an exercise program. Some patients with heart disease (for example, patients who have acute myocarditis, or an infection of the heart) should not undertake an exercise program until their problems are under control.

Exercise Prescription

The recommended program for people with coronary artery disease includes aerobic exercise, strength training, and stretching.[26] For most people, aerobic activity should begin with 5–10 minute periods and gradually increase to 30 continuous minutes on three non-consecutive days per week. There is strong evidence that this prescription decreases the likelihood of a second heart attack and increases the time that a person with classic angina pectoris can exercise before chest pain begins. Strength training has been found to be helpful in decreasing the symptoms associated with coronary artery disease and improving vitality. Appropriate warm-up and cool-down stretching should also be part of the program. Any regimen should avoid aggravating other problems that may be concurrent, such as osteoarthritis. If a particular exercise causes pain, discontinue it.

A guideline for creating an individualized exercise prescription is described in the ACSM's "Exercise for Patients with Coronary Artery Disease"[27] and includes mode, frequency, duration, intensity, and progression. The mode of aerobic training should include large muscle groups and continuous exercise such as walking, jogging, bicycling, or swimming. Strength training should include a series of 10–12 exercises (technically called circuit training) that are gradually added to the repertoire, initially in one set of 12 repetitions. Weights can be added and eventually two sets of 10 repetitions per set are performed. The frequency of endurance (aerobic) exercise should be at least three non-consecutive days per week combined with two to three days per week of strength training, and the duration should last for about 30–45 minutes. The intensity of the aerobic exercise should be between mild and moderate and approved by your doctor. It should not provoke an episode in which the heart receives insufficient blood or experiences an arrhythmia. The level of exercise that avoids these problems can be determined during the formal graded exercise stress test (performed before beginning a training program). The duration of aerobic training should be 20–40 minutes per session accompanied by 10 minutes of warm-up and cool-down stretching. The progression of the program should be slow and individualized by working with a professional.

Osteoarthritis and Increasing Range of Motion

Osteoarthritis is a degenerative disease that involves the breakdown and loss of cartilage in the joints and affects at least 20 million people in the United States.[28] Symptoms include pain, stiffness, and swelling in the joints and other supporting structures of the body, and the risk increases with age. Given the fact that osteoarthritis involves soreness of the joints, one might think that exercise would be contraindicated. However, the National Institute of Arthritis and Musculoskeletal and Skin Diseases (NIAMS) recommends not only that arthritic patients exercise, but that they include it in their comprehensive treatment program.[29]

NIAMS recommends "range of motion" exercises to maintain joint movement, relieve stiffness, and increase flexibility; strengthening exercises; and aerobics to improve cardiovascular fitness, help control weight, and improve overall function. "Range of motion" is the normal amount joints can be moved in a certain direction. See the Arthritis Foundation website (www.arthritis.org) for illustrations. Arthritis patients should consult with their doctors or physical therapists regarding which exercises are safe and effective. NIAMS recommends that range of motion exercises be done daily or at least every other day; strengthening exercises should be done every other day (unless there is severe pain or swelling); and endurance exercises should be done for 20–30 minutes three times a week (unless there is severe pain or swelling).

Like other individuals, osteoarthritis patients can exercise too much. If you have unusual fatigue, increased joint swelling or weakness, decreased range of motion, or pain that lasts more than an hour after a workout, you have exercised too much. If you experience any of these symptoms, decrease the duration or intensity of exercise.

Obesity, Weight Loss, and Exercise

Recent studies have found that the majority of people in the United States (66%) are either overweight or obese.[30] As explained in Chapter 6, body mass index (BMI) is a simple way of determining whether or not people are overweight. The normal BMI for men and women is 18–24.9, overweight is 25–29.9, and obese is 30 or higher. Methods used to determine overweight and obese children and adolescents take into account their changing height and development over time. Usually, growth charts are used and children and adolescents over the 90th percentile in terms of weight are considered overweight or obese. These conditions are associated with an increased risk of Type 2 diabetes mellitus, hypertension, heart disease, musculoskeletal problems, and a variety of other serious illnesses. Various public health agencies (including the Centers for Disease Control) and the Surgeon General are calling for a course of action to help the youth of our nation lose weight and keep it off. Although many people are now on weight loss programs, the majority of these diets fail. However, exercise programs added to a reduction diet may be a way of preventing obesity or maintaining needed weight loss once it is achieved.

For weight loss, exercise has several advantages over dieting, and a general improvement in fitness is helpful even if weight is not lost.[31] Also, increasing physical activity to achieve fitness is a more reasonable goal than weight loss and can be more easily recognized as an achievement. For example, if a person needs to lose 100 pounds, it can seem like a daunting task. On the other hand, if small increases are made in physical activity, that person will experience a rewarding improvement in vitality and energy.

For people who are obese, even small weight loss can result in significant improvements in many symptoms of certain chronic diseases, like diabetes mellitus or coronary artery disease. Exercise, in association with modest changes in diet, can result in improved blood sugar control or lessen some symptoms of coronary artery disease, such as chest pain (angina pectoris). Sometimes motivation can be achieved by monitoring laboratory tests associated with chronic illness. For example, moderate exercise programs can decrease hemoglobin A1c levels in diabetes mellitus (which is beneficial) and moderate exercise may reduce lipid levels in people at risk for coronary artery disease.

The National Weight Control Registry (www.nwcr.ws) is a group of over 5000 people who have successfully maintained a 30-pound weight loss for a year or more. Researchers have studied members to determine what contributed to their success[32] and learned that many had made unsuccessful dieting attempts in the past. Perhaps the most important factor that led to their ultimate success was learning to exercise almost daily, usually up to 60 minutes per session, checking their weight once a week, and being careful about caloric intake. Of course, it can take weeks or months of gradual increase and continued dedication to work up to regular exercise sessions of 60 minutes. An additional finding is that maintaining a normal weight appears to be more difficult in people who have a history of obesity than in people who have never been overweight.

Considerations for Eating Disorders Patients

There is no patient group in this chapter for whom the recommendation of exercise is more controversial than those with eating disorders—specifically anorexia nervosa and bulimia nervosa. Many, if not most, of these eating disorder patients engage in unhealthy exercise. As explained in Chapter Three, anorexics often suffer from activity anorexia, and exercise can be considered a type of purge for bulimics who binge and then try to burn off the calories by excessively exercising. Some healthcare professionals believe that moderate exercise is beneficial for nearly everyone—except severely emaciated individuals—and that it is virtually impossible to prevent eating disorder patients from exercising unless they are physically restrained or are being watched continuously. Thus, part of treatment may have an exercise prescription to allow the healthcare providers more control. However, many experts suggest that allowing or recommending exercise for this group of individuals is not only unhealthy from a medical standpoint, but that it borders on being irresponsible and unethical. Additionally, they add, a strong need to exercise has been associated with relapse.[33] Although many intensive treatment programs still prohibit exercise or activity, many others incorporate carefully planned, implemented, and monitored activity as part of the treatment regimen.[34]

To determine the appropriateness of exercise for someone with an eating disorder, several issues must be considered. Each individual differs in terms of his or her medical consequences, psychiatric diagnoses, medications, menstrual status (for women), weight, metabolism, the role of exercise in the disorder, treatment compliance, progress in treatment, and a host of other variables. Thus, decisions have to be made case-to-case.

Sometimes, it is "healthier" not to exercise. For example, anorexics should abstain from aerobic activity until they have maintained prescribed weight gain. Younger patients, especially athletes, need to be supervised, and parents can find excellent exercise guidelines in *The Parents Guide to Eating Disorders.*[35] Clinicians can find additional information in the appendix of *The Clinical Manual of Eating Disorders,*[36] but some helpful suggestions are provided here.

> Eating disorder patients must examine and change their attitudes and beliefs about exercise.

Eating disorder patients must examine and change their attitudes and beliefs about exercise. To begin with, they should receive information on "healthy" exercise that puts an emphasis on the role of good nutrition. Clarifying the varied purposes of physical activity—health, enjoyment, and sport—helps to show that it has value other than just losing weight. The dysfunctional relationship between exercise and eating must be changed so that patients stop using exercise as a way to compensate for eating. Instead, eating must be viewed as necessary to fuel exercise.

Patients must be taught how to increase body awareness while decreasing body obsessiveness. They need to listen to their bodies, recognize physical signals (i.e., pain, fatigue, hunger, etc.), focus on positive changes in how their body feels and what it is able to do, and to experience these changes as positive.

Further, patients must be assisted in satisfying needs previously met by, or associated with, unhealthy exercise. To do this, therapists commit to helping patients determine which functions, purposes, and needs were previously served by exercise, and devise healthier strategies for satisfying those needs in ways that are unrelated to exercise.

When reintroducing exercise to the eating disorder patient, several strategies are recommended. It must be determined by the treatment team that exercise will not increase the patient's risk. The patient should weigh at least 90% of expected weight, be progressing in treatment, be willing to increase caloric intake to account for an increase in activity, and be able to exercise "non-symptomatically" (not use exercise for weight maintenance or loss). In the beginning, exercise should tend toward resistance training and flexibility rather than aerobic, which burns more calories. Strengthening exercises can be particularly valuable because they provide the patient with an increased sense of emotional, as well as physical, strength. The duration should be brief, approximately 15–20 minutes, no more than one time per day, and be limited to 3–5 times per week. The intensity should be kept to no more than 60% increase of maximum heart rate, and should not occur for at least two hours after eating. If these initial strategies prove to be successful—the patient maintains a healthy weight and does not become obsessive about calories or working out—then the frequency, duration, and intensity can be increased and aerobic activities can be allowed.

Chronic Mental Illness and Exercise

Much less is known about the value of exercise for people with chronic mental illness, such as schizophrenia, bipolar disorder, major depression, or post-traumatic stress disorder. As explained in Chapter 6, these people are more likely to be sedentary and apt to develop related complications, such as obesity, diabetes mellitus, and hypertension. A number of factors contribute to this increased risk including symptoms of the illnesses themselves. For example, people with schizophrenia may be suspicious of others and afraid to leave their homes. Those with post-traumatic stress disorder may be easily startled and therefore less likely to go to the gym or participate in activities with others. People with depression may have low energy levels and sometimes multiple physical complaints that decrease the likelihood of exercise. Furthermore, as documented in a large study from Australia,[37] people with a mental illness are often from lower socioeconomic classes and have less access to exercise programs.

Individuals with serious mental illnesses are usually much less active than the general population. One study found that among 234 people with mental illness, only 12% participated in vigorous exercise compared to 35% in the general population, and participation in light physical activity was reduced as well.[38] Another study found that death due to heart disease was nearly twice as high among the mentally ill.[39] People with chronic mental illness die at earlier ages, and at least part of this increased risk may be related to sedentary lifestyle.

Recently, the advent of newer psychiatric medications that have the side effect of weight gain—particularly those used for the treatment of psychotic disorders—has led to a renewed interest in exercise. Treatment programs that increase physical activity may reduce some symptoms of mental illness as well as improve vitality and general fitness. These improvements may also lead to weight loss and reduce some of the complications of obesity.

Mood and Depression

Among the various mental illnesses, the effect of exercise on mood and depression has been best studied. Several studies have evaluated the effect of physical training on mood in older adults who have not been diagnosed with depression. For example, moderate intensity strength training has been shown to improve mood and vigor and decrease anxiety in adults who were an average of 68 years of age[40] and not clinically depressed. However, the most impressive studies have been with individuals who have been diagnosed with clinical depression—those who exercised had reductions of symptoms similar to the effects of various psychotherapy interventions.[41, 42]

Another group of researchers found exercise to be more valuable than a medication.[43] They compared three treatments for clinically depressed adults: aerobic exercise alone, antidepressant (sertraline, known as Zoloft) alone, and a combination of aerobic exercise and antidepressant. After 4 months there were no significant differences among the three groups, although patients taking sertraline improved more quickly. However, after 10 months the exercise-only group had significantly lower relapse rates than the two groups receiving medication.

Schizophrenia

Patients with schizophrenia are at particularly high risk for obesity and the "metabolic syndrome," a constellation of clinical and laboratory findings that increase the risk of cardiovascular disease. The main features are: abdominal obesity (a measurement based on the circumference of the waist compared to the hip), elevated triglycerides and abnormal cholesterol levels, elevated blood pressure, insulin resistance, and certain laboratory markers.[44] One sizeable Norwegian study found that the metabolic syndrome was more than four times as common among young patients (average age 31) with schizophrenia than among the general population.[45]

Clinicians have been concerned about the weight gain that occurs with atypical anti-psychotic drugs (particularly olanzapine, or Zyprexa), and various approaches have been studied. An educational program aimed at increasing exercise and altering food choices resulted in only a very modest weight loss (less than one pound) in the treatment group, whereas a significant weight gain (nearly 10 pounds) occurred in the usual care group.[46] Programs utilizing various cognitive-behavioral strategies have also found modest improvements in physical activity and small decreases in weight. However, despite the improvements found in anxiety and mood, the core symptoms of schizophrenia were not affected by physical activity.

Seriously mentally ill patients are at least as willing as the general population to begin exercising and may derive more benefits, but the approach needs to specialized. Since schizophrenics are often suspicious of others, exercise programs for them should be coordinated through the patient's mental health providers. Certain types of exercise may be more appropriate for this group, for example running on a treadmill at home rather than jogging through city streets.

Other Mental Illnesses

Although there are fewer studies about exercise and other mental illnesses, there is some evidence that patients with post-traumatic stress disorder experience a reduction in their core symptoms as well as a reduction in anxiety and depression when they begin an aerobic exercise program.[47] In another study, patients who had recovered from borderline personality disorder (BPD) had higher physical activity levels and were less likely to be obese or have hypertension or diabetes mellitus[48] than the group still suffering with BPD. Across the board, most evidence points to the positive effects of exercise for mentally ill patients.

The Role of Physicians

Throughout this book, readers have been directed to consult with a primary care physician before beginning a physical activity program. But, is the physician prepared to assist you? Unfortunately, most medical schools do not teach future doctors about the benefits of exercise, offer courses on how to counsel patients on modifying their behavior, or require students to exercise. Despite courses on anatomy and human biology, medical students often learn little about applied kinesiology, the study of mechanics and anatomy in relation to human movement. According to the deans and directors of education[49] at 128 medical schools in the United States, few of their students knew much about exercise. The respondents thought that although a majority of their graduates could competently conduct an evaluation to determine whether or not a patient could begin an exercise program, they doubted that the doctors could properly address their patients' prescriptive needs. Only 10% thought their graduates could design an exercise prescription, and only 6% said that their medical school provided a core course addressing exercise testing and prescription.

However, there is evidence that change is occurring. For example, researchers in Hungary[50] evaluated the physical activity level of medical students and found that most do not think their personal lifestyles are healthy. In response to this finding, their medical school implemented a required physical education program that requires students to exercise two days a week for two hours per session. The administrators believe that if a doctor models a healthy lifestyle and also learns how to write an appropriate exercise prescription, patients are more likely to improve their activity levels. In an example closer to home, the dean of medicine at a university in Florida has begun to develop faculty-student exercise programs and built a state-of-the-art fitness center. Unfortunately, to date, it has rarely been used.

It is important for individuals with chronic illnesses to consult with their doctor before beginning an exercise program. Ask plenty of questions about specific situations and your physician's expertise regarding what physical activity would be appropriate. If the doctor is not fully informed, ask for a referral to someone who is. As stressed throughout this chapter, exercise is usually beneficial, but people with special needs also require knowledgeable guidance.

Notes

1. *last round of exercise.* Schneider SH, Amorosa LF, Khachadurian AK, Buderman NB: Studies on the mechanism of improved glucose control during regular exercise in type 2 (non-insulin-dependent) diabetes. *Diabetologia 26:*325-360, 1984.

2. *people with diabetes mellitus.* Schneider SH, Khachadurian AK, Amorosa LF, Clemow L, Ruderman NB: Ten-year experience with an exercise-based outpatient lifestyle modifcation program in the treatment of diabetes mellitus. *Diabetes Care 15:* Supppl. 4):1800-1810, 1992.

3. *described in detail elsewhere.* Devlin JT, Ruderman N: Diabetes and exercise: the risk-benefit profile revisited. In: Handbook of Exercise in Diabetes. Ruderman N, Devlin JT, Schneider SH, Krisra A (Eds). Alexandria, VA, American Diabetes Association, 2002.

4. *body weight and composition.* Bryner RW, Ullrich IH, Sauers J, et al: Effects of resistant vs. aerobic training with an 800 calorie liquid diet on lean body mass and resting metabolic rate. *J Am Coll Nutr 18:*115-121, 1999.

5. *complications physical limitations.* Albright A, Franz M, Hornsby G, et al: American College of Sports Medicine Position Stand. Exercise and type 2 diabetes. *Med Sci Sports Exercise 32:*1345-1360, 2000.

6. *and sets of 10-12 repetitions.* Sbanez J, Izquierdo M, Arguelles I, et al: Twice-weekly progressived resistance training decreases abdominal fat and improves insulin sensitivity in older men with Type 2 diabetes. *Diabetes Care 28:*662-667, 2005.

7. *suffer from hypertension (high blood pressure).* Hajjar I, Kotchen TA: Trends in the prevalence, awareness, treatment, and control of hypertension in the United States 1998-2000. *JAMA 290:*199-206, 2003.

8. *availability of tasty, high fat foods.* National High Blood Pressure Education Program Working Group on High Blood Pressure in Children and Adolescents. The Fourth Report on the Diagnosis, Evaluation, and Treatment of High Blood Pressure in Children and Adolescents. *Pediatrics 114* (2 Suppl 4th Report):555-576, 2004.

9. *greater risk of heart disease.* Kannel WB, Wolf PA, McGeeDL, et al: Systolic blood pressure, arterial rigidity, and risk of stroke. *JAMA 245:*1225-1229, 1981.

10. *blood pressure response to exercise.* Matthews CE, Pate RR, Jackson KL, et al: Exaggerated blood pressure response to dynamic exercise and risk of future hypertension. *J Clin Epidemiol 51:*29-35, 1998.

11. *risk of heart attacks and strokes.* American College of Sports Medicine Position Stand: Exercise and Hypertension. *Medicine and Science in Sports and Exercise 36:*533-553, 2004.

12. *Currently, lifestyle changes.* Khan NA, McAlister FA, Lewanczuk RZ, et al: The 2005 Canadian Hypertension Education Program recommendations for the management of hypertension: part II – therapy. *Can J Cardiol 21:*657-672, 2005.

13. *greater for those with hypertension.* Pescatello LS, Kulikowich JM: The after effects of dynamic

exercise on ambulatory blood pressure. *Med Sci Sports Exerc 33*:1855-1861, 2001.

14. *all cause mortality by 4%.* Whelton PK, He J, Appel LJ, et al. Primary prevention of hypertension: clinical and public health advisory from the National High Blood Pressure Education Program. *JAMA 288*:1882-1888, 2002.

15. *22 hours after exercising.* Ronda M, Alves J, Braga A, et al: Postexercise blood pressure reduction in elderly hypertensive patients. *J Am Coll Cardiol 39*:676-682, 2002.

16. *age, gender, and ethnicity.* Pescatello LS, Bairos L, Vanheest JL: Postexercise hypotension differs between white and black women. *Am Heart J 145*:364-370, 2003.

17. *further studies in this area are needed.* Kelley GA, Kelley KS, Tran ZV: The effects of exercise on resting blood pressure in children and adolescents: a meta-analysis of randomized controlled trials. *Prev Cardiol 6*:8-16, 2003.

18. *irregular heart beat, heart attack.* Shaper AG, Wannamethee G, Walker M: Physical activity, hypertension, and risk of heart attack in men without evidence of ischaemic heart disease. *J Hum Hyperten 8*:3-10, 1994.

19. *possibly sudden death.* Giri S, Thompson PD, Kiernan FJ, et al: Clinical and angiographic characteristics of exertion-related acute myocardial infarction. *JAMA 282*:1731-1736, 1999.

20. *FITT Principle.* Pate RR, Pratt M, Blair SN et al: Physical activity and public health: a recommendation from the Centers for Disease Control and Prevention and the American College of Sports Medicine. *JAMA 273*:402-407, 1995.

21. *as effective as continuous exercise.* Thompson PD, Crouse SF, Goodpaster B, et al: the acute versus the chronic response to exercise. *Med Sci Sports Exerc 33*:S438-S445, 2001.

22. *leading cause of death among Americans.* Clark LT: Issues in minority health: atherosclerosis and coronary heart disease in African Americans. *Med Clin North Am 89*:977-1001, 2005.

23. *can negatively affect exercise tolerance.* Lenz TL, Lenz NJ, Faulkner MA: Potential interactions between exercise and drug therapy. *Sports Med 34*:293-306, 2004.

24. *same activity before chest pains begin.* Clausen JP, Tm-Jensen J: Heart rate and arterial blood pressure during exercise in patients with angina pectoris: effects of training and of nitroglycerin. *Circulation 53*:436-442, 1976.

25. *increase in HDL-cholesterol.* Tran ZV, Brammell HL: Effects of exercise training on serum lipid and lipoprotein levels in post-MI patients. A meta-analysis. *J Cardiopulmonary Rehab 9*:250-255, 1989.

26. *strength training, and stretching.* Stone JA, Cyr C, Friesen M et al: Canadian guideline for cardiac rehabilitation and atherosclerotic heart disease prevention: a summary. *Can J Cardiol 17 Supp B*:3B-30B, 2001.

27. *"Exercise for Patients with Coronary Artery Disease."* American College of Sports Medicine. Exercise for Patients with Coronary Artery Disease. *MSSE 26*:3, 1994, i-v.

28. *20 million people in the United States.* National Institute of Arthritis and Musculoskeletal and Skin Diseases (NIAMS), 2002. What is Osteoarthritis? Available: www.niams.nih.gov/hi/topics/arthritis/oahandout.htm.

29. *their comprehensive treatment program.* National Institute of Arthritis and Musculoskeletal and Skin Diseases, 2002. Arhrtitis and Exercise. Available: www.niams.nih.gov/hi/topics/arthritis/arthexfs.htm.

30. *are either overweight or obese.* Overweight and Obesity At a Glance. Surgeon General U.S. Department of Health and Human Services. Available: www.surgeongeneral.gov/topics/obesity.

31. *even if weight is not lost.* Lee S, Kuk JL, Davidson LE, et al: Exercise without weight loss is an effective strategy for obesity reduction in obese individuals with and without Type 2 diabetes. *J Appl Physiol 99:*1220-1225, 2005.

32. *contributed to their success.* Mc Guire MT, Wing RR, Klem ML, et al: What predicts weight regain in a group of successful weight losers? *J Consult Clin Psychol 67:*177-185, 1999.

33. *been associated with relapse.* Strober M, Freeman R, Morrell W: The long-term course of severe anorexia nervosa in adolescents: Survival analysis of recovery, relapse, and outcome predictors over 10-15 years in a prospective study. *Int J Eat Disord 22:*339-360, 1997.

34. *part of the treatment regimen.* Calogero R, Pedrotty K: The practice and process of healthy exercise: An investigation of the treatment of exercise abuse in women with eating disorders. *Eating Disorders 12:*273-291, 2004.

35. Herrin M, Matsumoto, N: *The Parents Guide to Eating Disorders.* Carlsbad, CA: Gürze Books, 2007.

36. Powers P, Thompson R: Athletes and eating disorders; In J Yager & P Powers (Eds.), *Clinical Manual of Eating Disorders* (pp. 357-385). Washington, DC: American Psychiatric Publishing, Inc, 2007.

37. *large study from Australia.* Glover JD, Hetzel DMS, Tennant SK: The socioeconomic gradient and chronic illness and associated risk factors in Australia. *Australia and New Zealand Health Policy 1:*1-8, 2004.

38. *was reduced as well.* Davidson S, Judd F, Jolley D, et al: Cardiovascular risk factors for people with mental illness. *Australian and New Zealand Journal of Psychiatry 35:* 196-202, 2001.

39. *twice as high among the mentally ill.* Lawrence DM, Holman CD, Jablensky AV, et al. Death rate from ischaemic heart disease in Western Australian psychiatric patients 1980-1998, *British Journal of Psychiatry 182:*31-36, 2003.

40. *average of 68 years of age.* Tsutsumi T, Don BM, Zaichkowsky LD, Takenaka K, Oka K, Ohno T: Comparison of high and moderate intensity of strength training on mood and anxiety in older adults. *Percept Mot Skills 87:*1003-1011, 1998.

41. *various psychotherapy interventions.* Craft LL, Landers DM: The effect of exercise on clinical depression and depression resulting from mental illness: a meta-analysis. *Journal of Sport and Exercise Psychology 20:*339-357, 1998.

42. *various psychotherapy interventions.* Lawlor DA, Hopker SW: The effectiveness of exercise as an intervention in the management of depression; systematic review and meta-regression analysis of randomized controlled trials. *British Medical Journal 322:*763-767, 2001.

43. *more valuable than a medication.* Blumenthal JA, Babyak MA, Moore KA: Effects of exercise on older patients with major depression. *Arch Intern Med 25:*2349-2356, 1999.

44. *and certain laboratory markers.* Grundy SM, Brewer HB, Cleeman JI, et al, for the Conference Participants. Definition of metabolic syndrome. Report of the National Heart, Lung, and Blood Institute/American Heart Association Conference on Scientific Issues Related to Definition. *Circulation 109:*433-438, 2004.

45. *among the general population.* Saari KM, Lindeman SM, Viilo KM: A 4-fold risk of metabolic syndrome in patients with schizophrenia: The Northern Finland 1966 Birth Cohort Study. *J Clin Psychiatry 66:*559-563, 2005.

46. *occurred in the usual care group.* Littrell KH, Hilligoss NM, Kirshner CD, et al: The effects of an educational intervention on antipsychotic-induced weight gain. *J Nurs Scholarsh 35:*237-241, 2003.

47. *aerobic exercise program.* Manger TA, Motta RW: The impact of an exercise program on post-traumatic stress disorder, anxiety, and depression. *Int J Emerg Ment Health 7:*49-57, 2005.

48. *have hypertension or diabetes mellitus.* Frankenburg FR, Zanarini MC: The association between borderline personality disorder and chronic medical illnesses, poor health-related lifestyle choices, and costly forms of health care utilization. *J Clin Psychiatry 65:*1660-1665, 2004.

49. *deans and directors of medical education.* Connaughton AV, Weller RM, Connaughton DP (2001). Graduating medical students; exercise prescription competence as perceived by deans and directors of medical education in the United States: implications for Healthy People 2010. *Public Health Reports 116:*226-234.

50. *researchers in Hungary.* Angyan L (2004). Promoting physical activity in medical education. Mini-review. *Acta Physiol Hung 91:*157-166, 2004.

Index

About the Authors

Pauline Powers, MD is a professor of psychiatry and behavioral medicine at the Health Sciences Center, University of South Florida. She has been treating patients with obesity and eating disorders for over 30 years and currently runs the Eating Disorder Program at Fairwinds Residential Treatment Center. She has been involved in integrating moderate exercise programs into the treatment of patients for years, including people with severe obesity, anorexia nervosa, and bulimia nervosa. She was the founding president of the Academy for Eating Disorders and is a past president of the National Eating Disorders Association. Recently she was a member of the American Psychiatric Association Work Group on Eating Disorders that prepared the *Practice Guideline for the Treatment of Patients with Eating Disorders,* 2006. She has also coauthored *Athletes and Eating Disorders* with Ron Thompson, which appeared in the *Clinical Manual of Eating Disorders.*

Ron Thompson, PhD is a psychologist in private practice, specializing in the treatment of eating disorders. He has been a consulting psychologist for the Athletic Department at Indiana University-Bloomington for the past 20 years. In addition to his clinical work, Dr. Thompson lectures, writes, and conducts research on the topic of eating disorders, as well as provides education and training regarding eating disorders to athletes, coaches, and other sport personnel and healthcare professionals at NCAA member institutions. Most recently, he has coauthored the Disordered Eating section of the International Olympic Committee Medical Comission Position Stand on the Female Athlete Triad and the *NCAA Coaches Handbook: Managing the Female Athlete Triad.* Included in his publications are the books *Helping Athletes with Eating Disorders* and *Bulimia: A Guide for Family and Friends.*

About the Publisher

Since 1980, Gürze Books has been dedicated to providing quality information on eating disorders recovery, research, education, advocacy, and prevention. They also publish books on related topics, such as exercise, self-esteem, body image, and health at every size. Their websites include www.gurze.com, which is a comprehensive resource on eating disorders, and their blogsite: www.eatingdisordersblogs.com.

To Order

The Exercise Balance is available at bookstores and libraries and may be ordered directly from the publisher, Gürze Books. Quantity discounts are available.

The company's website is a comprehensive resource about eating disorders. It features books and free articles on the subject and related topics including exercise, self-esteem, body image, health at every size, and more. It also has links to eating disorders nonprofit associations and treatment facilities. Their resource catalogue is handed out by thousands of therapists, educators, and other health care professionals around the world.

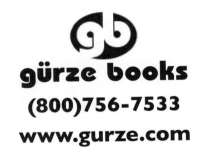

gürze books
(800)756-7533
www.gurze.com